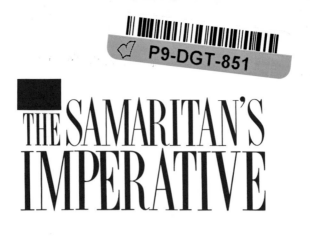

THE SAMARITAN'S IMPERATIVE

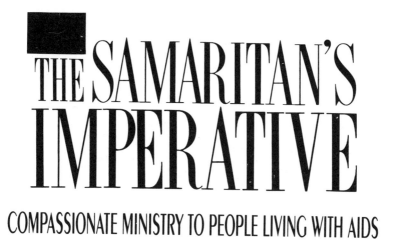

THE SAMARITAN'S IMPERATIVE

COMPASSIONATE MINISTRY TO PEOPLE LIVING WITH AIDS

Michael J. Christensen

ABINGDON PRESS

Nashville

The Samaritan's Imperative:
Compassionate Ministry to People Living with AIDS

This book is printed on acid-free paper.

Unless otherwise noted, scripture taken from the HOLY BIBLE, NEW INTERNATIONAL VERSION. Copyright © 1973, 1978, 1984 International Bible Society. Used by permission of Zondervan Bible Publishers.

All Scripture quotations marked RSV are from the Revised Standard Version of the Bible, copyrighted © 1946, 1952, 1971, 1973. Used by permission.

All Scripture quotations marked KJV are from the King James Version of the Bible.

Back cover photograph of Joey Benko and Michael Christensen by Greg Schneider.

Library of Congress Cataloging-in-Publication Data

Christensen, Michael J.
   The Samaritan's Imperative: compassionate ministry to people living with AIDS / Michael J. Christensen
     p. cm.
   ISBN 0-687-36790-5 (alk. paper)
   1. AIDS (Disease)—Patients—Pastoral Counseling of. 2. AIDS (Disease)—Religious aspects—Christianity. 3. Church work with the sick. I. Title.
BV4460.7.C466 1991
259'.4—dc20
                                  90-47212
                                      CIP

MANUFACTURED IN THE UNITED STATES OF AMERICA

Acknowledgments

Significant ministry is never the result of individual effort, but community involvement. I wish to thank the members of the AIDS Mission Group, which was initiated in 1987 by Golden Gate Compassionate Ministries in San Francisco, for their support of and involvement in the completion of this project. Many of the AIDS stories embedded in the text were written and contributed by mission group members who are themselves AIDS caregivers, including Rebecca Laird, Bonnie Wong, Muriel Beukelman, Carl Stuart, Tom Cahill, and Jack Pantelao. Barb Rost (whose brother died of AIDS) and Susan Foley (my soul friend) also contributed a story to the project.

I want to thank those who feverishly reviewed and wisely edited my manuscript: my gifted wife, Rebecca Laird, and my loyal friends Steve Worthington, Michael Dotson, Jim Rutz, and Paul Moore.

I am particularly indebted to my supervisor at San Francisco General Hospital, the Reverend Connie Hartquist, director of the Episcopal Chaplaincy, who has tried to teach me by word and example *the ministry of presence.*

I am also grateful to my District Superintendent, Clarence Kinzler, who has defended me in controversy and reminded me that the church is "neither pro-gay nor anti-gay, but anti-sin and pro-people." It was he who challenged me to "find a way to walk the line between acceptance of persons and endorsement of life-style" in ministry to gay persons with AIDS.

Finally, to my beautiful daughter, Rachel Laird Christensen, born when I was completing this manuscript, I gratefully dedicate this book. When death and dying are all around me, she reminds me of the hope and new life we have in God.

Contents

Preface

A Personal Pilgrimage in AIDS Ministry

Every ministry has its roots. My personal pilgrimage in AIDS ministry began in San Francisco in the spring of 1983, two years after the AIDS crisis began in the United States. Although I had read newspaper and magazine accounts of a growing epidemic among homosexuals, I never expected to find a person with AIDS in my path. I was fully involved as pastor of Golden Gate Community Church and as director of a homeless mission, Golden Gate Ministries. AIDS was simply not my issue or calling.

Then Malcolm contacted me one day, desperate to talk with a Nazarene pastor and make peace with God and the church of his childhood. He had left the Nazarene church after college, moved to San Francisco, and eventually contracted AIDS. The day he came to see me in my office was the beginning of AIDS ministry for me.

I was uninformed about AIDS and unresolved in my attitude toward homosexuals. But I knew the Good Samaritan story, and realized I must respond to the person in my path. Malcolm's inspiring story of reclaiming his Christian faith, reuniting with his church and family, and dying in his mother's arms is told in chapter five.

In 1984, I was contacted again by a former church member infected with HIV. Peter had just tested positive and was running scared. He feared that AIDS was God's punishment for his homosexual life-style. In counseling him, I challenged his view that AIDS was a punishment sent from God. In my words and actions, I tried to represent the God of grace and mercy, "slow to anger and abounding in steadfast love." I tried to help Peter understand that God does not "treat us as our sins deserve or repay us according to our iniquities. . . . For as a father has compassion on his children, so the Lord has compassion on those who fear him" (Ps. 103:8-13).

Kneeling in prayer at the sofa in my office, Peter confessed his fear of retribution and need for grace and healing. He reaffirmed his faith in Jesus Christ and committed to live for God. The following Sunday he was in church with a desire to be part of the Christian community. Peter became our church pianist, and he and his roommate hosted a weekly Bible study in their home. Slowly, I was learning how to respond to HIV disease.

In 1984, I had the privilege of traveling to India, meeting Mother Teresa, and working in her home for the dying. At the entrance to Kalighat, Mother Teresa's home for the dying in Calcutta, a sign reads: "THE GREATEST AIM IN HUMAN LIFE IS TO DIE IN PEACE WITH GOD." The Missionaries of Charity simply offer loving attention in the name of Jesus, nurturing a dying person back to health or helping that person die with dignity as a child of God. "We let the one who has lived like an animal die like an angel," says Mother Teresa.

I remember hand-feeding a frail young woman who was very close to death. She had pitting edema, and when I pressed her arm a permanent indentation was left. We managed to hook her up to an intravenous line of medication that prolonged her life for a few days. She was in tremendous pain. She died, but not alone. She was surrounded by Mother Teresa and her sisters and volunteers, who stayed with her for the duration. My work in India at the home for the dying prepared me for hospice work in San Francisco. In 1985, I served as a chaplain-on-call at a community hospice center. On Sunday afternoons, several of us from Golden Gate Community Church conducted a hospice service for those with a life expectancy of six months or less. The hospice movement values loving care and empowerment of terminally ill patients. Success is to die in peace and dignity, ideally at home, and if at all possible, in the company of those they love. Most of the hospice patients I visited died in peace and dignity and in the loving presence of friends and family. This is not the case in most hospitals where death is viewed not as a community event or spiritual transition but as a private matter and a medical failure.

In 1986, Charles, one of our homeless clients at the mission I directed, was diagnosed as having AIDS, and applied for residency at Golden Gate's Oak Street House. (The Oak Street House, founded in 1981, is a home for the homeless and those in transition and recovery, sponsored by Golden Gate Compassionate Ministries in San Francisco.) Charles had been married and had two children, but over the years he had lost touch with them. He was a drug addict and a drifter. Our residency program was intended to house the homeless in transition, but was not equipped to provide health care services to an applicant with AIDS. We were able to get him admitted to a shelter for people with AIDS and later into the hospital, and managed to stay in touch with him in the course of his disease.

Condemning Charles for using dirty needles was not called for; he knew better than we did that AIDS was the result of his years of drug abuse. Our ministry was to withhold judgment and support him in completing his life before he died. Charles made courageous gestures toward reconciliation with his family, attempting unsuccessfully to contact his former wife and children. He sent his love to friends at the mission. He read the Psalms in the wee hours of the night, and prayed and sang with those who came to see him. He struggled with issues of faith and forgiveness, mortality and spirituality. At joyful moments, he found peace with God, himself, and others. At angry moments, his disposition dispelled his peace of mind and heart.

When he finally died in the hospital of three AIDS-related opportunistic diseases, the only family the hospital knew to call was the staff at Oak Street House. We claimed his body and arranged his funeral. Charles's funeral was the first AIDS service that I officiated. A group of his homeless friends and mission group members gathered to say good-bye. I recounted some of the details and significance of Charles's life and death. Others shared remembrances of how he struggled in life. "I love you guys!" were his last words to those who had faithfully supported him, listened to his story, and witnessed to God's presence and love.

The following year, in the fall of 1987, one of our Sunday school kids, six-year-old Joey Benko, was diagnosed with AIDS. How shocking for us to discover that AIDS afflicted not only gay men and drug addicts, but also children who received blood transfusions tainted with HIV.

Golden Gate Community Church was not a large church. But in the six short years since the inception of the epidemic, two gay men, a drug addict, and now a child with AIDS had literally shown up at our door. It was imperative to respond, regardless of the cost involved, through compassionate ministry.

Beyond starting a church and mission sponsored AIDS

ministry called the BRIDGE (the full story of which is told in chapter 5), I personally enrolled in a twelve-week program called "AIDS Ministry Training for Religious Professionals" through the Episcopal Chaplaincy at San Francisco General Hospital. After graduating, I became a chaplain on the AIDS ward and outpatient clinic.

My first year as an AIDS chaplain radically changed my life. One of the first issues I was forced to deal with was my fear of possibly catching AIDS. Despite the reassurances from medical researchers that the risk of HIV infection apart from its known means of transmission is minimal, I harbored unnecessary fears. What if I accidentally got stuck with a contaminated needle left in a hospital trash can, or touched the bleeding body of an AIDS patient? I reminded myself that Jesus did not call us to a completely safe life. Rather, he called us to count the cost of discipleship and risk all for the kingdom.

Studying the response of the ancient church to plagues in Rome helped me, and I prayed for radical trust in God and healthy abandonment to compassionate ministry. William Barclay, in his commentary on Philippians, reminds us how the early church engaged in high risk ministry in time of plague:

> In the days of the early Christian Church there was an association of men and women called the *parabolani,* the "gamblers." It was their aim and object to visit the prisoners and the sick, especially those who were ill with dangerous and infectious diseases. In A.D. 252, plague broke out in Carthage; the heathen threw out the bodies of their dead, and fled in terror. Cyprian, the Christian bishop, gathered his congregation together and set them to burying the dead and nursing the sick in that plague-stricken city; and by so doing they saved the city, at the risk of their lives, from destruction and desolation. There should be in the

Christian an almost reckless courage which is ready to gamble with his life to serve Christ and to serve men. The Church always needs the *parabolani*, the "gamblers" of Christ.[1]

The second issue that challenged my outlook was the moral implications of AIDS. Drug abuse and sexual promiscuity are known factors in the risk of AIDS, and ministering to people with these life-styles is controversial. While there is a place for "tough love" in recovery from addictive behavior, and moral concern in AIDS prevention, I have chosen to emphasize the *unconditional love and acceptance* of the gospel. Before the church can moralize and confront sin in a person's life, it must first become a healing agency of God's grace and forgiveness to those who are struggling. Judgment and condemnation are never called for in the church's mission; understanding and support are in keeping with the call.

I try to walk the line between acceptance of persons and endorsement of life-style. To offer unconditional love and acceptance of persons is not to imply moral agreement or to license sin. To refuse to judge people and the ways they have chosen to live their lives is not to "wink at sin" or deny moral standards.

Yet attempting to walk the line, I have found, results in raising suspicions on both sides of the fence. Liberals shout "homophobia" or "moralism" in response to talk about the moral implications of AIDS, while conservatives cry "pro-gay" or "soft on drugs" to a withholding of judgment of sinful life-styles. Though a difficult path to walk, there is a middle ground that recognizes moral standards for AIDS prevention while offering nonjudgmental ministry to

1. William Barclay, *The Letters to the Philippians, Colossians, and Thessalonians*, The Daily Study Bible (Philadelphia: Westminster, 1959), pp. 62-63.

persons living with AIDS, who do not need our prescriptive judgments or moral condemnation.

Whenever I feel caught in the middle, in the cross fire of this controversy, I have found great solace in the words of Martin Luther: "Here I stand, I can do no other." For readers who prefer a more definitive position either endorsing or condemning certain activities and life-styles, I offer a challenge: *Don't let your passion for a cause prevent you from having compassion for people!*

The Samaritan's Imperative offers a nonjudgmental approach to AIDS ministry based on biblical principles and personal experience. Although intended as a practical guide, it reviews some of the moral and theological issues raised by AIDS and points to the story of the Good Samaritan as the model for compassionate response.

The Samaritan's Imperative is divided into two parts: (1) how to withhold judgment and respond with compassion; and (2) how to become a care-giver. Embedded in the chapters are short stories about persons with AIDS and their caregivers. I hope that these stories give the reader a feel for the day-to-day realities of living with AIDS.

In my previous book, *City Streets, City People,* I included a chapter entitled "AIDS—the New Leprosy." *The Samaritan's Imperative* takes up where that chapter left off, and shows how any church or individual can start a compassionate ministry to people living with AIDS, regardless of how they were infected.

Although anyone can become infected with the AIDS virus, most of the people I visit as a chaplain are gay persons with AIDS. This has caused me to apply the biblical principles of compassionate ministry more to gay persons with AIDS than to the other high risk groups. For this imbalance, I apologize.

I have written this book for mothers and fathers, sisters

and brothers, of persons living with AIDS. I have written for ministers and laity in the church, knowing that families who have been touched by AIDS are in every congregation. I have written for those called by God to AIDS ministry, knowing it will take a vast network of compassionate care-givers to respond to the needs of people living with AIDS.

Like the ancient Samaritan walking down the Jericho road, confronted by a person in need, there is a *Samaritan's Imperative* for Christians and all people of goodwill to follow their consciences and respond to need.

For me, *The Samaritan's Imperative* is a deeply personal journey of faith, one that has called me away from places of comfort and clarity into disturbing pioneer territory, leaving no presupposition unchallenged. AIDS ministry for me has been a journey of discovery, filled with unbelievable surprises and rewards that come from trusting God for provision and wisdom. I hope the reader catches a glimpse of the joy and fulfillment available in an otherwise intense and somber service of compassionate ministry.

It is to this high adventure in compassionate ministry that the reader is invited to embark.

PART ONE

RESPOND WITH COMPASSION

CHAPTER ONE

Walking Through the AIDS Ward

"I hate it when they stick me. I can't stand it. Last time, she stuck me five times before getting it in. I just don't want to go through it all again."

As an AIDS chaplain in San Francisco, I'm in contact with a diverse group of people who have one thing in common—HIV disease, better known as AIDS. Weekly I walk through the AIDS wards at San Francisco General Hospital, which serves approximately two thousand outpatients and forty inpatients with HIV (human immuno-deficiency virus). My colleagues and I find it one of the most intense and challenging ministries imaginable.

I invite you to walk with me through the valley of the shadow of death, and allow me to tell you of four persons who are representative of thousands living and dying with AIDS. I then want to reflect with you about how terminal patients come to life at death's door, and how no one should have to die alone.

WARD 86

The elevator opens onto the eighth floor of the 125-year-old original red brick building known as San Francisco General Hospital. Ward 86, the AIDS Clinic, is teeming with activity as outpatients try to keep their monthly appointments. The clinic, cheerfully and tastefully decorated, is a warm and friendly place, even if it is overly crowded.

There are basically two locations on Ward 86 to visit with outpatients: the waiting room, where making eye contact is necessary to find someone who wants to talk; and the treatment room, where patients are waiting to see their doctor or receiving transfusions or drug therapies.

I walk into the treatment room and see a thin black man lying on a bed covered with his coat. Approaching him, I ask: "Mind if I sit down for a visit?" He seems grateful.

George tells me it had been a "year of hell" since his diagnosis. Halfway through his story, a nurse walks over and prepares to put an IV in his arm for treatment. George panics. "I hate it when they stick me. I can't stand it. Last time, she stuck me five times before getting it in. I just don't want to go through it all again."

I offer to stay with him until the nurse hooks him to his line. George calms down, smiles, and says: "You are God's angel!"

I respond in kind: "The Lord sent me here today to hold your hand because God loves you so very much."

The nurse tries to take some blood samples. George, predictably, is a "hard stick." Unable to find a viable vein, the nurse says, "These arms feel like drug arms."

George admits he is a drug user. His arms are skin and bones and hard as rocks—the result of "overcooking" them with drugs. "I'll have to find a vein you haven't used very much," says the nurse, tightening the tourniquet. After several unsuccessful attempts, the nurse finally gets the needle in. George screams at the top of his lungs. I tightly hold his hand, hoping this ordeal will soon be over. Finally, the monthly procedure is complete. George and I have become friends and hope to see each other again. I leave the room to complete my rounds for the day.

"IT's As REAL As IT GETS AT SAN FRANCISCO GENERAL" reads the favorite staff t-shirt at General. General is where most of the city's poor, homeless, and uninsured patients go for medical treatment. If a derelict goes into withdrawal and is in medical danger, he or she is brought to General. If a drug addict overdoses, or a street person gets stabbed in a fight, or a poor mother is about to give birth to her baby, General is the hospital of last resort. And if a person with AIDS is not insured, General is the only place to go.

WARD 5A

On the fifth floor of the main building at General, a well-equipped, bright, cheerful, and model unit known as "5A" is filled with AIDS patients. An interdisciplinary team consisting of medical professionals, social workers, counselors, and chaplains is responsive to an ever-changing group of patients.

It is the chaplain's role to visit, listen, and help a patient spiritually prepare for life or death. Usually there are five chaplains covering the AIDS ward. Every day is covered except Saturdays.

One Saturday, a young man I'll call Skip lies dying on his bed. He is a difficult and demanding patient who has finally reached the final stage of a sad and sorrowful life. One of the growing numbers of homeless persons with AIDS, Skip has been a body builder, a con artist, an armed robber, and an IV drug user. Today, he is skin and bones and looks close to death. His arms are like hardened rubber from years of abusive injections. He is hooked up to seventy milligrams of methadone and wears an oxygen mask. His breathing is deep and erratic. He slips in and out of consciousness, and probably won't last the night.

Since no chaplains are on duty and no volunteers are available, the attending nurse tries calling friends and agency staff members who know him, trying to find someone to be with him in his final hours. Living on the streets, Skip has very few friends who could respond to a phone call. He had been staying downtown in a shelter for homeless persons with AIDS, but no one there had time to come and see him.

Skip knows he is dying and wants to go quickly. He manages to pull off his oxygen mask, gasping for breath. The nurse quickly replaces it. He takes it off again when she leaves the room.

Death does not come soon. Several hours later Skip dies, alone.

Every week people die on the AIDS ward. According to the head nurse at the AIDS Clinic at General, "many patients die terrible deaths. Gasping as much as sixty breathes a minute, they often drown in their own fluids. They die of fevers, respiratory diseases, cancers, and dementia. AIDS is the ugliest kind of death I've seen!"

Usually family or friends are with patients when they die. But not always. No ONE SHOULD HAVE TO DIE ALONE!

To watch someone die of AIDS is to be confronted with utter helplessness. *What do you do?* You hold a hand. You say a prayer. You say good-bye.

How do you feel? You feel the life force wrenched away from its anchor in regions of the soul. You feel as if you are watching a gathering storm. You know in your heart that soon everyone will know someone who will die from AIDS. We will all feel the devastating impact of this modern-day plague.

"I JUST STOPPED BY TO SEE HOW YOU'RE DOING"

Again, I am walking down the hall of unit 5A, and I enter the room of Arlo, age thirty-nine, a tired and dying man. "Hello, my name is Michael, and I'm the chaplain on this unit. I just stopped by to see how you're doing." With these almost routine words, I manage an entrance rite. By finding a way to meaningfully ask the question "How are you doing?" you'll find that most patients are willing to tell you their story.

Arlo tells me he grew up as a Roman Catholic, but after getting married, he joined an evangelical fellowship in San Francisco. He tells me of his blood transfusion in 1985 and about his devoted wife and family. "God only knows; God only knows," he says repeatedly about why he now has AIDS. Arlo is from Haiti and speaks in broken English in simple sentences through an oxygen mask. I tell him I know his pastor and ask about his faith in God. He tells me of his recent prayers of devotion and his fears of dying. I try to assure him that his spiritual strength will carry him through. After an hour, I say good-bye and leave the room. I wash my hands and commit Arlo to God, praying that in my absence, God will draw near with peace and presence.

The following week, I return to visit my friend Arlo. He is drifting in and out of consciousness. The sound of fluid in his lungs and his deep, erratic breathing through his oxygen mask indicate that death is near.

Placing my hand on his chest and feeling the perspiration soaking through his gown, I pray for his troubled spirit. I anoint him on his brow in the Name of the Father, Son, and Holy Spirit and quietly pray for God to comfort him.

Arlo's wife, Jana, is present and she motions for me to follow her outside the room. She asks me if I think Arlo is holding on because of her and their children. I respond: "I don't know. Let's be sure we give him permission to go."

We go back inside and Arlo becomes alert. "Honey, are you in pain? Are you able to breathe?" Jana asks.

His eyes widen and he attempts to smile: "I'm all right."

As Arlo clutches his oxygen mask, gazing into Jana's loving, tearful eyes, I pray a prayer of affirmation and release. Gently rubbing his chest, which had become so thin, I attempt to say good-bye: "Arlo, the Lord loves you so much. Your family loves you too and thanks you for providing for them. We will all miss you. Your family will be okay. You can stay here with us as long as you wish, or leave us any time. Whenever you're ready, whenever the Lord calls, just go and reach for the Lord's hand."

Arlo points to the calendar on the wall. His brother, who has joined us, takes it down and brings it over to the bed. It has an idyllic picture of a mountain and a stream. Arlo is delighted by the scene, and we all comment on its beauty. "He has caught a glimpse of heaven," I suggest, "and is trying to show us what it is like."

I leave the room about 8:00 P.M. Before I leave the hospital for the night, I enter the chapel on the second floor and kneel before the barren cross above the altar. I pray for the patients I visited today, and ask that whatever healing is available—whatever comfort can be found, whatever family and friends are available—be brought to each in need. I try to leave patients in the hands of God, and not carry their needs home as a personal cross to bear. Although it is difficult, I know it is important to both commit them to God and to rest.

Jana and Arlo's brother remain with him all night long. Early the next morning, Arlo quietly dies, not alone but in the company of his family and connected to the source of his spiritual strength.

I thank God that Arlo did not have to die alone. I am outraged that others do! Not everyone who dies of AIDS has a loving family who will sit for hours by his or her side and pass the long and lonely days of approaching death. Not everyone who dies of AIDS makes peace with herself and her God.

Although chaplains make visits and do what they can,

and family members and friends respond as they are able, AIDS care-givers are needed across the land to bridge the gap and represent a God who loves and forgives and welcomes the weary home. NO ONE SHOULD HAVE TO DIE ALONE!

"I DON'T WANT TO SEE A CHAPLAIN!"

Another day presents new opportunities for ministry on the AIDS unit. I typically meet patients by knocking on a door, walking into a room, and saying the same words I said to Arlo: "Hello, my name is Michael, and I'm the chaplain on this unit. I just stopped by to see how you're doing." Most AIDS patients are happy to see a chaplain.

The room at the corner with a beautiful view of the city is Kevin's room. Kevin responds coldly to my introduction: "I'm not religious, and I don't want to see a chaplain."

"Now why is that?" I ask.

"Because I've had quite enough religion stuffed down my throat growing up. Thank you very much!"

"In what church were you raised?" I ask.

"Southern Baptist! But now my folks are Nazarene. They dragged me to church at Christmas time last time I saw them. It was pretty bad."

"Do your parents know about your diagnosis?"

"No, they don't, and I'm not going to tell them. If they knew, they would start praying for a deathbed conversion, and I'm not going to do that."

"You think your parents would have a hard time dealing with AIDS?"

"I think they would."

"Listen, Kevin, if you ever decide to tell them, and you need someone from their denomination to help them deal with it, I would be pleased to serve as your advocate. I'm a minister in the Church of the Nazarene, and I'm available."

Kevin seems surprised at my affiliation and thanks me for the offer. He writes down my name and phone number just in case.

A few months later Kevin is back in the hospital, and he has finally told his parents he has AIDS. They call me from Arizona and tell me their son is gay and is dying of AIDS. They want to come out to see him.

I try to prepare them for seeing their son. "Kevin knows how you feel about his homosexuality; you don't have to tell him again. He also knows how long you have been praying and hoping for him to come to Christ. You don't have to remind him. Why don't you *simply love him and accept him* as your son who is sick? No judgment, no scriptures to think about, no speeches on what he needs to do, just come and be with him."

They agree and tell me they had stopped sending him Gospel tracts and pressing for his salvation years ago. They are eager to see the son they love.

Kevin braces himself to see his parents by telling his friends that his parents are fundamentalists and might try to convert him. "They think unless you believe like them, you'll go to hell. Don't let them lay that on me, please! I don't want a deathbed conversion," he says emphatically.

His parents come to town to visit their son. True to their word, they are loving and accepting. They withhold any moral judgment that they might feel. It has been twenty years since their son left home and the church. It is devastating for them to see him in the hospital with AIDS. They stay for a few days and have to go home.

I return to the hospital to see Kevin after their visit. I ask him how the visit had gone. He is relieved and delighted. "They surprised me," he says, remarking on how supportive and accepting they were. "It was a good visit."

"Did they try to convert you?" I ask.

"No, they didn't."

I tell Kevin he is welcome to live in our Care House after he gets out of the hospital, if his doctor thinks it appropriate. He smiles and thanks me for the offer. Kevin is not released from the hospital but becomes progressively more ill. Some days he is coherent, and other days he is not. AIDS is literally destroying his brain. His doctor schedules him for a biopsy.

On the eve of Kevin's operation, Carl Stuart, a Baptist minister and fellow chaplain in the hospital, visits him. It is during this visit, that something happens deep within Kevin's spirit that he swore to his friends would never happen. His heart opens to Christ on his deathbed, as Carl Stuart explains:

"You Should See My View!"
by Carl Stuart

"You should see my view from my room," Kevin told his parents over the phone, between the sobs. Something wonderful had happened that changed his perspective on everything.

The view was exceptional that day from the AIDS Ward at San Francisco General. Through the familiar fog that gently embraced Twin Peaks shone a piercing sunlight in beautiful, powerful rays.

Kevin had been lying in spiritual darkness and the "shadow of death" for weeks. He had set his will against God as he understood God from his childhood. His experience with the evangelical church left him feeling rejected and angry. But God had called him "out of darkness and into his marvelous light" (I Pet. 2:9 RSV).

It was early evening when Kevin's partner approached the nurses' station with unopened letters to Kevin in his hand. The request from Kevin's parents was for Michael Christensen to open and read them to Kevin, and to support him through the emotional and spiritual impact the letters might bring. The letters were what might be the last words from two of his brothers who were unable to come in person.

Since it was not Michael's day to be at the hospital, I agreed to read the letters to Kevin. Before I opened the first letter, Kevin asked: "Could we pray first?" We bowed together and prayed for courage of heart and strength of spirit to hear what was to be said.

The first message was inscribed on a card: " . . . there is NO ONE quite like you!" And proceeded to urge his brother to accept God's love.

Kevin broke into tears as we attempted to get through the passionate words from his brother.

The other letter followed. It exuded love and doctrine as he carefully cited the Scriptures he wanted his brother to consider. "All are sinners, not because of the sins they have committed, but because of the nature which they have received at birth," he wrote. But "God hath given us eternal life. And this life is in his Son. He that hath the Son hath life. And he that hath not the Son of God hath not life" (I John 5:11 KJV).

As the words of life continued to flow from the letter, it was not yet evident that the Spirit of Grace was caressing Kevin's heart, warming his soul for the seed that had been planted in childhood.

Time passed as we stopped again and again for Kevin to cough, to cry, to consider. At the end of the readings, I asked Kevin how he would like to respond to his brothers. By letter? By phone?

Again he said, "I want to pray." Without prompting, Kevin uttered a faltering but sure expression of saving faith: "God, I want to ask you into my life. . . . I'm sorry it has taken me so long."

I reminded him of Paul's words, "Therefore being justified by faith, I have peace with God through our Lord Jesus Christ" (Rom. 5:1 KJV).

The crying stopped, the countenance changed, the courage came to call his parents to tell them his good news. We dialed, they answered, and he said, "I have accepted Jesus, and he has given me such peace." And then came the tears of joy, the kind that only can come from heartfelt gratitude to God for the gift of Peace.

No wonder the view from Kevin's room was different. As he looked out the window and saw the setting sun pierce through the fog on the hills of Twin Peaks, it was as if he was seeing a place prepared for him in heaven. As he pointed out to me the area at the foot of the Peaks where he lived, I knew he saw far beyond to his final home. Facing the imminent brain surgery, for which he had prepared for three days, he exclaimed, "You should see the view from my room!"

Kevin went into surgery the following day, and physically took a downward turn. Two weeks later he lay unconscious in the loving presence of his sister and his partner of fifteen years. Their last words to him constitute an important though sorrowful good-bye: "Kevin, you can go home now." Permission granted, Kevin is free to die, if that is his wish. In that very moment, Kevin leaves this life behind, finally free from his season of pain. Because of courageous friends and family members, Kevin did not have to die alone!

Kevin made peace on God's terms, not his parent's or the church's. He returned to Christ on his deathbed, and told God, "I'm sorry it has taken me so long." Not exactly the modern evangelical formula for conversion, but it fits the truth of how people come to life at death's door.

COMING TO LIFE AT DEATH'S DOOR

When people ask me why I'm attracted to ministry with those who are dying, I answer: "Because that's where life happens!" People who know that they are dying seem more willing to deal with life, finish their work, and make peace with God. As Saint Bernard is quoted as saying: "Life is only for love. Time is only that we may find God."

How do terminally ill patients find God? How and why does a person on the threshold of death open up to God's love and presence? What's going on beneath the surface of conscious confession and conversion? Does God's Spirit speak more deeply to the human spirit when death draws near?

When I worked with Mother Teresa and her sisters in their home for the dying in Calcutta, I witnessed a kind of pre-confessional conversion, an almost unconscious receptivity to God's love and forgiveness in a number of poor and dying persons. I noticed that some, after many days of harboring anger, despair, and pain, opened their hearts to the love of the sisters and found peace and joy before they died.

They did not verbally repent or confess their faith in Jesus Christ. But below the surface, in the realm of the spirit, they were responding in faith to the God who loved them and desired to take them home. The truth shone forth in their eyes and was written on their faces. Mother Teresa and her sisters simply discern in the spiritual countenance of the dying the grace of God. The sisters believe that when the dying patients open up to God's love, they belong to God as much as if they had made a formal confession or verbal profession of faith.

I see the same process in AIDS ministry—terminal patients coming to spiritual life at death's door despite any lack of verbal confession, baptism, or communion.

A conscious and verbal profession of faith is essential for living in a community of faith, but it may not be necessary for one who is dying and responding to God. "Deep calls to deep" (Ps. 42:7), and "the Spirit searches all things, even the deep things of God" (I Cor. 2:10).

If saving faith is fundamentally a spiritual encounter, it should not surprise us that AIDS patients and other terminally ill persons respond to God from the depth of their being as they prepare to die and return to their Creator. We should not expect detailed, precise confessions of orthodox belief from such "deathbed conversions." The eyes themselves are adequate windows of the soul in touch with God. Any verbal testimony or theological reflection on the faith experience is helpful, but not essential as death draws near.

NO ONE SHOULD DIE ALONE

Walking through the valley of the shadow of death, you meet all types of people and see all kinds of needs. No one is beyond hope or should have to face AIDS alone.

The majority of AIDS patients in San Francisco still are gay or bisexual men. In central Africa, AIDS is primarily a heterosexual disease. Sexually active people who engage in unprotected intercourse continue to be at risk for AIDS worldwide. Historically, sex is not a subject the church feels comfortable discussing and therefore tends to condemn or ignore those who contract AIDS through sexual contact. This makes understanding AIDS doubly difficult. But sociological and moral objections should not stand in the way of offering compassionate care to terminally ill people. We have learned to respond appropriately to cancer patients; we don't ask how much they smoked or about their diet as they face death. We simply offer compassionate care. Can we not do the same with AIDS patients?

Increasingly AIDS patients are IV drug users. People who stick dirty needles in their arms are at the highest risk for AIDS worldwide. Society and the church have a difficult time feeling compassion for those who intentionally abuse their bodies. But consider this: In Mexico, South America, and other countries people often inject their medication and share needles. To make matters worse, clinics in the Third World often cannot screen blood, sterilize syringes, or take precautions that are now routine in North America and most of Europe. Whether by abuse or misuse, those who most of contracted AIDS through contaminated needles need our love and understanding, not our judgment.

Sometimes persons with AIDS are children born to infected mothers, or born prematurely, requiring transfusions before the blood supply was safe. The number of HIV-positive infants and young children with AIDS is growing at an alarming rate. It is projected that by 1992 one out of ten pediatric beds will be filled by a child with AIDS. Most people have compassion for children with AIDS, yet the mothers and fathers of these children, who are often drug users or who had intercourse with an infected partner, need our compassion too!

AIDS, whether contracted out of medical ignorance, sexual carelessness, or drug abuse, is tragic and forgivable. When someone you know has AIDS, withhold judgment and respond with compassion. No human being—regardless of how a person got the disease—should be left to face it alone!

I continue to walk through the valley of the shadow of death, not alone but in the company of others. Together, we sense the breath of God blowing on the AIDS wards and outside the hospital. God is working behind the scenes, in the homosexual, minority, and heterosexual communities, among IV drug users, and in the lives of children. Healing happens even when there is no permanent cure. People respond to God and come to life at death's door.

The AIDS epidemic represents an extraordinary time in human history and calls for extraordinary measures to save the human race. The kind of response that is needed is the Good Samaritan's compassionate response. My friend and fellow AIDS care-giver Jack Pantaleo tells a story of compassion about two monks walking back to their monastery in the freezing cold:

AIDS—A Family Matter
by Jack Pantaleo

As they cross a bridge, two monks hear a man calling for help in the ravine below. They want to stop, but know they must reach the monastery before sunset or they will freeze to death.

The first monk chooses to risk the danger of the cold in order to help another to safety. He climbs down into the ravine and gathers the wounded man into his arms, and slowly makes his way back to the monastery.

The second monk has already gone on ahead, determined to get back safely before sunset.

Night comes, and with it the bitter cold.

As the first monk nears the monastery, he stumbles over something in the middle of the road. To his sorrow, it is the body of his brother who had gone on alone and had frozen to death. In seeking to save his life, he had lost it.

But the compassionate monk, willing to lose his life, was kept warm by the heat exchanged from carrying the stranger in need.

May we, in helping each other in the time of AIDS, save ourselves.

CHAPTER TWO

Back to Basics—Love, Acceptance, and Forgiveness

"I'm not a religious person. Why would God want to help me now that I'm sick? I never asked him for anything in all my life, and now it's too late."

Jesus told a powerful story about a man who had two sons whom he asked to go and work in the fields. The first son responded, "No, I will not go," but later changed his mind and went. The second son responded, "Yes, I will go," but later changed his mind and did not go.

"Which of these two did what his father wanted?" Jesus asked the chief priests and elders of the people. "The first one," they answered.

"I tell you the truth," said Jesus, "the tax collectors and prostitutes are entering the kingdom of heaven ahead of you!" (Matt. 21:28-31 paraphrased).

I have seen some of the most unlikely people (by religious standards) responding to the compassion of Jesus. Drug addicts, male and female prostitutes, and homosexuals shunned by society and the church are coming to faith in God. Some Christians seem upset, as if more is required in salvation than coming to Christ *just as I am*. This observation brings me back to the basics—the simple gospel of *love, acceptance, and forgiveness*[1] as the essentials of faith.

---

[1]Jerry Cook and Stanley Baldwin wrote a book by this title *Love, Acceptance and Forgiveness* (Ventura, Calif.: Regal Books, 1979) to help equip the church to be inclusive and non-judgmental. I am grateful to them for reminding me and others of the radical simplicity of the gospel of Jesus Christ.

THE GOSPEL IN A WORD IS LOVE

In the Old Testament, the law of love was understood only to apply to friends and family. Levitical law forbade Israelites from taking revenge or bearing a grudge against one of their own people. They were to overlook faults and "love your neighbor as yourself" (Lev. 19:18). Jesus practiced and taught an ethic based upon Judaic values, yet with a twist: "You have heard it said 'Love your neighbor, hate your enemy.' But I tell you to love your enemy, do good to those who hate you, bless those who curse you, turn the other cheek, give up your coat, go the second mile, do unto others what you would have them do unto you" (Matt. 5:43-48; Luke 6:27-36).

Jesus redefined *love* and applied it to everyone. Love was not just a blood bond or an emotional connection to family and friends. Love, for Jesus, was a radical willingness to be merciful even to those you don't like; a deep compassion that desires the best for others, even those who hate you; an indiscriminate expression of concern for friend and enemy alike. Love genuinely wishes a person well, demonstrates good will, is kind and courteous, returns good for evil, whether one feels like it or not.

"If you love only those who love you," Jesus says, "so what? Even tax collectors do that! And if you are good only to those who are good to you, big deal! Everybody does that. But if you love your enemies, if you are merciful to those who are guilty, if you love your neighbor as much as you love yourself, then there is merit. You have really fulfilled the law of love."

Does this mean that we are to love persons with AIDS as much as we love ourselves? Even if we think they are getting what they deserve? Is the homosexual my neighbor? The drug addict? The AIDS-infected mother who gave birth to a baby with AIDS?

35

The Samaritan's Imperative

A certain attorney, an expert in Jewish law, asked Jesus, "Who is my neighbor?" In response, Jesus told him a story of a man who was mugged on the road to Jericho and left in a ditch to die. Two religious leaders—a priest and a Levite—stumbled over the injured man and did nothing. Perhaps they thought this particular person was outside the scope of God's concern, or perhaps they were too busy with other professional priorities. Consequently, a person was left to die alone.

Finally, a Samaritan came by and showed compassion to the man in the ditch. Maybe it was because he, as a Samaritan, knew how it felt to be ignored as an outcast. Maybe it was because he understood the compassion of God. Whatever the motivation, this Samaritan took the injured man to a place of safety and care—the very thing he would have wanted for himself, if he were the man in the ditch.

Jesus, after telling this story, turned the question around. "Which of these was the neighbor to the unfortunate man?" The lawyer responded, "The one who showed compassion." Jesus said, "Go and do likewise" (Luke 10:25-37).

There are two striking truths in this story: First, Jesus intentionally chose a Samaritan as a model of loving compassion. We must note that the term *Good Samaritan* would be as much a contradiction to first-century Jews as *good lesbian* would be to many people today.

Orthodox Jews were taught to despise their neighbors in Samaria. After all, they had intermarried with other races. They were not careful to keep the whole law. They refused to worship in the Temple in Jerusalem, preferring their own sanctuary on Mount Gerizim. The disciples asked Jesus to pray down God's judgment on wicked Samaria (Luke 9:54), for Samaritans were to be avoided at all costs (John 4:9). Could not Jesus have picked a safer, less offensive example to teach neighborly love? Why did he have to speak so positively about a disobedient, discredited, outcast group? Perhaps it was to shock his audience and thus enlighten prejudicial consciences. Making the hated Samaritan the hero and the respectable priest and Levite the villains in the parable would be like having the "good lesbian" save the victim while the preachers and other prominent persons deserted their own.

Undoubtedly, Jesus shocked his audience in order to make the point clear that *how you treat people in need is more important than social and religious respectability.* Even the most despised and rejected of persons can be better neighbors than those who claim to be God's people.

A second striking truth is that Jesus did not define *neighbor* in terms of geographical proximity, religious compatibility, or sociological sameness. He did not say that only a person who lives in the *right* place, believes the *right* things, behaves the *correct* way, or is sexually oriented in the *proper* direction could be a neighbor. What he said was that *the person in need is my neighbor, and I am a neighbor when I help someone in need.* And if I am ever in need, I might be more than a little surprised to find out who my neighbors are.

Jesus shrewdly turned the lawyer's question around from "Who is my neighbor?" to "Am I a being neighborly?" There is no us versus them in this kind of love. We are not to love from a position of superiority but of mutuality. We are not to help the less fortunate with an air of paternal pity or condescension, but with a humble spirit of concern for our neighbor in need. *Neighbors helping neighbors* is what Jesus taught.

How shall we apply Jesus' teaching of loving your neighbor as yourself to the AIDS crisis? We do not have to look any farther than to the folks next door. How do good neighbors normally treat each other? Well, you find out who lives next door or upstairs or across the hall. You learn their names and listen to their stories. You are cordial, kind, and friendly. You invite them over for dinner or dessert. You freely lend them a cup of sugar or a stick of butter, if they ask. You compare notes on life and politics and religion. You express interest in how they are doing. You ask about their kids or family. You show up in moments of crisis and celebration. If the folks next door act in a morally objectionable manner, you don't condemn, but rather seek to understand. And when it is appropriate, you talk about your faith in God.

I commend one of the early members of our AIDS Mission Group, Bonnie Wong, as an example of a good neighbor. She never imagined becoming involved with AIDS patients but desired simply to work behind the scenes in a supportive role. Yet she was the first one in our group to have a neighbor diagnosed with AIDS.

Neighbors
by Bonnie Wong

I live in unit 317 and Joseph lived in unit 349 in a condominium complex in the heart of the city. We met about three years ago when he moved in, and we quickly became friends, especially after an emergency incident in our building to which we both responded.

In every neighborhood association, there are those who sit quietly on the sidelines and allow others to do the work. And there are those who pitch in and help where needed. Joseph was a neighbor who took an active part in the maintenance needs of our building and made himself available. Later, when his physical condition weakened, he would still volunteer for jobs when others would not. About two years ago, both Joseph and I found ourselves limping around the building. I was suffering from an injured knee, and he said he had a sore foot. I found out later, when I asked him how he was doing, that he had AIDS. He had not told anyone else, but wanted someone in the building to know, so he chose me. I felt honored by his trust but shocked and saddened by the diagnosis. I did not want my friend to die! (Someone later asked me if I knew how Joseph got AIDS, and whether or not I had confronted him about his life-style. In the light of impending loss, it did not seem a relevant point. I simply wanted to help.)

When the opportunity came on Thanksgiving Sunday to attend an AIDS healing service at Metropolitan Community Church, I wanted to invite Joseph. I was hesitant and had to overcome my usual social shyness. I reminded myself that my neighbor had AIDS and that I was inviting him out of friendship and concern.

The plan was to meet at the Oak Street House for prayer and then proceed to Metropolitan Community Church for the service. Joseph accepted my invitation and accompanied me to the house. During the prayer time, he shared with the group why he came: "I don't do church. But I do trust Bonnie, because she's my friend."

I felt that his affirmation was due to God rather than to anything I could take credit for. He was welcomed by our group with open arms, and we offered to pray for him. He said, "Okay."

Our District Superintendent, Clarence Kinzler, who joined us for the prayer time and the service, told Joseph that he could trust this group to support him. We all gathered around Joseph as Pastor Kinzler prayed with the laying-on of hands. I'm sure he felt the overwhelming love of God. At the healing service that followed, many more were prayed for in the same manner and with the same results.

Thanksgiving passed and Christmas time arrived. I invited Joseph to go Christmas caroling with our group. He was not able to make it, but expressed his appreciation in a kind note. He also asked me to keep him in my prayers.

A Christmas contribution of $265 for the needs of people with AIDS came to our mission group from some of the staff members at Harper & Row Publishers, where one of our members worked. Fifty dollars was entrusted to me to use for Joseph's benefit. When I tried to present it to him as cash, he refused. Only after considerable coaxing did he accept it for tickets to the Kirov Ballet.

In the course of our friendship, I had been praying for an opportunity to talk with Joseph more clearly about my faith in God. One night, a fire broke out in an old historic building a block away from our condominium. As huge flames jumped up into the night, Joseph and I watched the fire together. He told me he was ready to tell his parents that he was gay and that he had AIDS. This was a major step. I asked him if he wanted me to pray for him. He replied: "I was hoping you would say that."

I believe that there is a mustard seed of faith when people ask for prayer. Although Joseph was raised Catholic, he said his parents' religion had not impacted him much. But now he was thinking about God and prayer.

His first conversation with his parents went very badly, he said. But in the following week he received more positive support from them. His medical condition changed drastically in the spring.

When I returned home from church one Sunday afternoon, I saw an ambulance in the driveway. My denial was strong, and I refused to admit that Joseph might be dying. He was being assisted into a wheelchair and was going to the hospital. I called out his name. He looked up briefly, said, "Hello, Bonnie," then dropped his head. I did not know it at the time, but that moment was the last I would see him.

Joseph got weaker after he entered the hospital. Kaposi's Sarcoma had affected his stomach. Since he was unable to receive oral medication, he was given morphine intravenously. He managed to hold on until his parents arrived. He died peacefully the very next day.

Joseph's death reminded me of the brevity of human life and how precious is our daily health. It also taught me that God brings unexpected people into our lives for a reason. These are divine appointments, and we either grasp them in the moment or else let them slip away.

The ministry of love and acceptance is so important. It didn't seem like I did much for Joseph, but I was there for him when he called. Perhaps simple friendship is the most important gift we can offer to our neighbor in need, especially if our neighbor has AIDS.

Is the person living with AIDS in my city or yours as much our neighbor as the friend next door? Does the fact that a person with AIDS may also be a gay, a drug addict, sexually promiscuous, or a hemophiliac make him or her any less our neighbor?

These are important questions, not to answer but to live with. It is sometimes easier to play it safe and leave our neighbor dying in the ditch rather than offer him support. It is sometimes easier to clutch our robes of righteousness and pass by on the other side of the road in order to avoid guilt by association if our clothes should get dirty. And it is always more difficult to see the "sinner" as the model of a good neighbor than the more easily respected "saint."

The challenge of compassion is to see ourselves as a neighbor on the same level as our neighbor in need. Only as we overcome the divisive we-they mentality can we exchange real compassion with our good neighbors.

LOVE ACCEPTS EVEN THOUGH IT MAY NOT APPROVE

There will always be people who are difficult to love and accept. They may be homosexuals, AIDS patients, drug users or, conversely, Moral Majority types. But unless a person in need of love feels understood and accepted by another, any change of heart or life-style will be impossible. The gospel challenges us to be unconditional in our love and accept people *just as they are*.

What does *acceptance* mean? A pastor from my childhood taught me early in life the principle of unconditional love and acceptance: "Love accepts even though it may not approve! Love believes the best about a person, even if I do not agree with the choices a person makes. Love supports a person even though it may not sanction a particular action."

Unconditional love is more than the traditional principle of "love the sinner but hate the sin." Loving the sinner while hating the sin is a well-meaning attempt to separate a valued person from despised behavior, but is unlikely to succeed. Scripture reminds us that sin is not purely behavior but proceeds from the heart. Hatred of sin implies judgment of the sinner. Better to love and accept the whole person unconditionally, than to try to love the part that is not sinning.

Acceptance Means Loving Yourself

The gospel is such good news that it's difficult to believe. It goes against our basic notion that we must perform, produce, straighten up, and get it right in order to be loved and accepted. I think that is why many people prefer a gospel of works to a gospel of grace. We are not comfortable with unconditional love.

Trusting in a God who believes in us brings health and wholeness to our broken lives. This same trust makes it possible for us to love and accept others.

We can offer our neighbor unconditional love and acceptance only to the degree that we are able to love and accept ourselves unconditionally. Self-love and acceptance come with the knowledge that God loves and accepts us *just the way we are!* The good news is that God is *for us* and not against us, that we are invited to feast at God's table *without first changing in order to be worthy* of God's love. We are already loved, understood, and accepted by the God who created us in the divine image.

Since the divine image in every person is tainted by sin, we are personally challenged and made free to respond, grow, and change as we let ourselves be completely loved by God. The process begins with the divine invitation to come "just as I am" and does not end until we are completely reconciled. The changes in character and behavior that accompany Christian growth and disciple-ship are brought about by God alone, in God's time and way, and cannot be imposed or prescribed by others. We can support each other, and we can also hold each other spiritually accountable in living moral and compassionate lives. But we must not judge each other.

Acceptance Means Withholding Judgment

Jesus said, "Judge not, that you be not judged. For with the judgment you pronounce you will be judged, and the measure you give will be the measure you get. Why do you see the speck that is in your brother's eye, but do not notice the log that is in your own eye?" (Matt. 7:1 RSV).

The Apostle Paul reiterates this principle in his litany of sins in Romans 1. After listing every vice and idolatry imaginable, including "shameful lusts" and "indecent acts," he ends the passage with these words of warning: "You, therefore, have no excuse, you who pass judgment on someone else, for at whatever point you judge another, you are condemning yourself, because you do the same things" (Rom. 2:1).

43

Why are we not content to leave judgment and mercy in the hands of God? What is it that compels us to play God by judging our neighbor?

Judgmentalism is actually a defense mechanism that protects us from despising in ourselves what we see in others. The judgmental tendency allows us to project on others something that we ourselves feel guilty about. We thus find a scapegoat. When we judge or condemn another, we distance ourselves from God and reject others. This is why untold evil is done in the name of truth and righteousness, replacing a gospel of grace and freedom with a doctrine of prescription and conformity.

Judgmentalism never helps a person find forgiveness and healing; it only sends a message of disgust and rejection. People with AIDS especially feel the judgment of society. They quickly divide their world into those who accept them and those who reject them. When we, as care-givers, are judgmental, however subtly, we lose effectiveness in ministry. Just as professional counselors must learn to be nonjudgmental when relating to clients, so also AIDS care-givers must learn not to judge those whose values and choices are at odds with our own.

Acceptance Means Associating with "Sinners"

The measure of nonjudgmental, loving acceptance is how freely we mix and associate with people who do not share our values. Do we have friends outside the church? Are we invited to parties and events that the self-righteous would avoid? Do we have homosexuals as friends? Are we afraid to help alcoholics or drug addicts? Do we dare socialize with people with AIDS whom society shuns and stigmatizes?

Jesus ruined his reputation by associating with the "sinners" and outcasts of his day. He loved and accepted

Gentiles and Samaritans; he defended prostitutes and tax collectors; he ate and drank with gluttons and drunkards; he healed lepers and the sick. Jesus was not concerned about "guilt by association."

AIDS care-givers, likewise, tend to be identified with those they seek to help. Members of society, as well as representatives of the church, will wonder about your motives, perhaps even suspect you of being homosexual, using drugs, or having AIDS. They will have a difficult time understanding why you are involved in ministry with "those kind of people."

By befriending social outcasts, Jesus demonstrated that the kingdom of God included those Israel rejected. The way Jesus loved and accepted "sinners" on their own turf is best displayed by his conversation with the Samaritan woman at Jacob's well (John 4). The episode is a model for the kind of nonjudgmental, compassionate acceptance called for in AIDS ministry.

Jesus and the Woman at the Well

Tired and thirsty from his journey through Samaria, Jesus sat down by Jacob's well. When a Samaritan woman came to draw water, he asked her for a drink. She was surprised that Jesus even acknowledged her presence, for Jews did not associate with Samaritans.

"If you knew who asked you for a drink," said Jesus, "you would ask him for a drink, and he would have given you living water."

"Sir," the woman said, "the well is deep and you have nothing to draw with. Where can you get this living water?"

Jesus answered: "Everyone who drinks this water will be thirsty again, but whoever drinks the water I give will never

45

thirst. Indeed, the water I give will become a spring of water deep inside, welling up into eternal life."

The woman said to him, "Sir, give me this water."

It was *after* Jesus offered her living water that he inquired about her living situation: "Go, call your husband."

"I have no husband," she replied.

"You are right when you say you have no husband. The fact is, you have had five husbands, and the man you are living with is not your husband. What you have said is true."

"Sir," the woman said, "I can see that you are a prophet."

Reflecting on this passage, we can note that this woman was considered an outcast for at least three reasons:

1. She was a *Samaritan*, and Samaritans were despised by the Jews because they broke the law, worshiped in the wrong place, and intermarried.

2. She was a *woman*, and women were considered property, not persons, and treated at best as second-class citizens in Israel. According to Rabbinic teaching, every Jewish male was enjoined to pray each morning, thanking God that "He did not make a Gentile, . . . a woman, . . . or a boor" (*Talmud Tos Berakoth*).

3. She was a *rejected* woman. In Jesus' day, men could easily divorce their wives for any reason, but wives could not leave their husbands. This woman had been rejected by five husbands, and the man she now lived with wouldn't even marry her! Jesus was not condemning this woman for divorce or for living in sin, he was simply letting her know that he understood her rejection and why she lived the way she did. Jesus was not at all judgmental, and the woman's response was not defensive. She recognized that Jesus was a prophet.

The point of the story is that Jesus offered this woman unconditional love and acceptance, the very gift she was seeking.

I Know You Are Thirsty

I know a "Samaritan" woman who has three strikes against her: (1) she has *AIDS*—a terminal disease with a cruel stigma; (2) she's a *woman* with AIDS, which makes the social stigma even harder to deal with; and (3) she is *addicted* to drugs—a desperate way to live. Her name is Jewel.

She was sitting upright on the bed and appeared to be crying when I visited her in the hospital. Walking into her room, I said, "Are you okay?" She said that she was fine, just a little infection in her eyes.

Jewel looked a mess—disheveled hair, her eyes oozing, a rash on her face and arms, missing a few teeth, her body very thin. I've seen street prostitutes and IV drug users with this same desperate appearance at General.

She recognized me as a chaplain and invited me to come in. I noticed a picture of Jesus on the wall and a Bible and rosary beads on the table. "Are you Catholic?" I asked.

"Not really," she replied. "I don't go to church. But after I got diagnosed, I contacted a priest, and he baptized me with water. He also gave me a Bible."

"Have you been reading it?"

"Well, I've tried. But I have trouble understanding it."

"What book are you reading?" I asked.

"Revelation."

"Why don't you start at the front rather than at the back?"

"That's what the priest told me to do, and he said not to read Revelation. But that got me interested in what's in there."

"Would you like me to read you a couple of paragraphs?" I asked.

"Sure, that would be great," she said.

So I opened up her Bible and began reading in Revelation 21.

Then I saw a new heaven and a new earth. . . . And I heard a loud voice from the throne saying, "Now the dwelling of God is with men and women, and he will live with them. They will be his people, and God himself will be with them and be their God. He will wipe every tear from their eyes. There will be no more death or mourning or crying or pain, for the old order of things has passed away."

I paused to see if Jewel was still with me. Tears were dropping from her eyes. Whether or not she understood the meaning of the passage, the truth of the images spoke deeply to her heart. I skipped to chapter 22 and continued reading:

Then the angel showed me the river of the water of life, as clear as crystal, flowing from the throne of God and of the Lamb down the middle of the great street of the city.

I stopped reading and asked, "Can you picture a flowing river in the middle of Market Street?"
"Oh yes!" she said with delight.

On each side of the river stood the tree of life, bearing twelve crops of fruit, yielding its fruit every month. And the leaves of the tree are for the healing of the nations.

"Imagine that, Jewel," I said excitedly. "The river of God flowing right down Market Street, with life-giving trees on the banks yielding fruit for food and leaves for healing!" She was as intrigued as I was with the image of a God who loved us so much to provide a river connecting our needs with the resources at the foot of God's throne.

Jewel's joy was mixed with sorrow as she told me of her two daughters, ages four and ten, who would be left alone when she died. She was worried about them, and wondered if God would take care of them. I said I believed God would bring someone into their lives to love them as much as she did, and that God would not abandon them or leave them alone.

She then shared with me part of her story of rejection and abuse, and how she stopped using drugs only to find out that she was infected. She questioned God's wisdom in allowing so much suffering in the world. And again, she cried for her children.

I was with her in her pain for about an hour. I listened carefully and reminded her of God's love, acceptance, and forgiveness. I also told her of God's gift of strength in time of need. It was obvious that she was a woman of prayer, holding on against great odds to the single strand of faith that was hers. The good news was almost too good to believe—that God understood, believed in her, and wanted to provide for her children.

Before I left, I offered a blessing. Tears filled her tired, anxious eyes. I knew in my heart that Jewel was drinking "living water" from the River of God, which would make all things new.

FORGIVENESS ON GOD'S TERMS, NOT OURS!

Forgiveness is the most difficult gospel ingredient to understand and freely receive from God. As one who has been steeped in church tradition, I wonder if we, the church, have put restrictions on God's grace? Perhaps we should rethink our doctrine of divine forgiveness.

How do modern-day "sinners" find forgiveness in the church? Universalists make it easy: God is Love, and Love is God. Love means everyone is already saved. You don't have to repent. Guilt is a negative emotion. You don't have to be forgiven, you just have to forgive yourself! Visualize your potential. Think positive. Be free.

Moralists make it difficult: God is Love, but God is also holy and righteous and hates sin! Before the good news, there is bad news. You're a sinner. You're bound for hell. You need to repent. So come to *our* church and get saved. If you're living in sin, you must get married or move out. If you're gay, you must be celibate or get help in changing your orientation. If you're attending the "wrong" church, you must come to the "right" one. To believe the right things and do the right things is to be forgiven.

The problem with liberal "universalism" is that grace is cheap, evangelism useless; there are no ideals to live up to, and it costs nothing to follow Christ. Yet Jesus said it would cost everything; we must deny ourselves to follow him.

The problem with traditional "moralism" is that grace is restricted, and salvation requires a submissive relationship with the organized church, or a view of the Bible that prescribes exactly *what to do* and *what to believe*.

There is a more moderate and biblical position between these two extremes. If we turn to the example of Jesus in the Gospels for an understanding of grace and forgiveness, we are immediately struck with his departure from orthodox doctrine and prescriptive morals.

According to the orthodoxy of Jesus' time, if you were a Gentile and wanted to convert to the Jewish religion, there was a prescribed method of conversion: You had to submit to circumcision (however painful), promise to obey the Laws of Moses as interpreted by the elders (however unreasonable), and agree to worship God in the Temple in Jerusalem (however distant).

If you were a Jewish sinner and wanted to be forgiven, you had to present yourself before the chief priests and offer an acceptable sacrifice at the Temple. Only priests could hear your confession, and pronounce you clean. Once you were cleansed, you were forever obliged to conform to the prescribed laws and ceremonies of Israel. Some sins, like sodomy and adultery, were generally punishable by death. Some persons, like lepers and eunuchs, were hopelessly outcast and denied access to the community of faith. And some, like prostitutes and tax collectors, were so despised that even if they did repent, no one would believe or accept them. How did such "sinners" who came to Jesus find forgiveness? In blatant contradiction to ancient Jewish orthodoxy, Jesus not only loved and accepted them just as they were, but he also forgave them before they asked or fully recognized him as the Messiah.

Throughout the Gospels we see that Jesus' understanding of repentance and forgiveness was radically different from that of his Jewish heritage. While strict Judaism offered inclusion only to the carefully religious and self-righteous, Jesus received "sinners" into the kingdom before they had properly repented according to the prescribed method. The kind of repentance he recognized in the "sinner" was an inner brokenness and humility of heart. The kind of faith sufficient to bring forgiveness was an openness to the love of God. Jesus would look into a person's heart and pronounce the "sinner" clean and already "forgiven."

A Sinner's Love

Jesus was "no respecter of persons" and was willing to dine with anyone. As described in Luke 7, it was a Pharisee who had invited him to dine when a woman came with an alabaster jar of expensive perfume and knelt weeping at Jesus' feet. She began to wash his feet with her tears and wipe them with her unbound hair. Then she kissed his feet and anointed them with perfume.

51

Since this woman was in the house of the Pharisee, he had to know her. Still, he feigned shock and surprise at her appearance and said: "If this man were a prophet, he would know what kind of woman this is!" As everybody knew, this was a bad woman, a sinful woman with unbound hair, a harlot. Characteristically, Jesus did not condemn her. Instead, he recognized in her brokenness and gratitude that she already had been forgiven. If she had not desired salvation and wholeness, if God had not granted her forgiveness and healing, she would not have been kneeling and weeping at his feet.

Jesus said to his host: "I came into your house—you gave me no water to wash my feet. This woman has washed my feet with her tears and wiped them dry with her hair. You did not welcome me with a kiss, but she has not ceased kissing my feet. You did not anoint my head with oil, but she has anointed my feet with perfume! I tell you the truth, her many sins are forgiven."

The principle of forgiveness that Jesus revealed was this: *The one who has been forgiven much loves much. The one who has been forgiven little loves little.* The Pharisee presumably kept the law and did not sin. Therefore he felt no need for forgiveness, and his love was shallow. The sinful woman, on the other hand, was conscious of her need, and was overwhelmed to the point of tears. Her love for Jesus was deep. The one who loves much is forgiven much, for generous love is the sign of deep forgiveness. The one who loves little is forgiven little, and reveals through self-righteousness the shallowness of grace in one's life.

If there is a hierarchy of sin, then the worst sin must be Pharisaism—living in denial, deception, self-righteousness, and self-sufficiency. The greatest sin is to be unconscious of sin in your life. But even the smallest sense of need will open the gates to divine forgiveness. To the woman who loved deeply, Jesus said: "Your sins are forgiven. Your faith has saved you. Go in peace" (Luke 7:48, 50). Suppose the sinner in this story were a flamboyant gay man with AIDS? You are the host, and Jesus is the guest. Can you see Jesus offering this man love, acceptance, and forgiveness on the same terms as the "sinful woman?" Perhaps this man is a male prostitute. Perhaps he has used drugs to numb the pain of life. Perhaps the fact that he has AIDS has made him receptive to divine love and forgiveness. What do we say to this man with a dreaded disease? What do we do when he starts to cry uncontrollably when Jesus embraces him and calls him friend? Do we see in his eyes the brokenness of his life? Do we discern in his words and demeanor a quality of character that reveals a wrestling with his Creator? Do we judge by his outward appearance, or do we look upon the heart?

To withhold judgment and respond with compassion brings the healing presence of God. This is the essence of AIDS ministry.

It's Never Too Late

I met Earl on the morning after he was officially diagnosed with AIDS. He was understandably anxious and upset. I asked him how he felt. He said he felt sad.

"It's been thirty-five years of hell and now this . . ."

"Now what?" I asked.

"My life has been so bad up till now and then to top it off with AIDS is . . . I don't know. I have lots of regrets—the drugs, the street life."

"Would you like to tell me your story? I bet you've been through a lot."

53

Over the next hour, Earl told me his life story, which included never knowing his father, sexual abuse by his stepfather, criminal activity and incarceration as a youth, the early death of his mother, running away from home at sixteen, surviving on the streets of San Francisco, hustling for money as a prostitute, IV drug use, cruel and exploitive relationships, loss of lovers, and now AIDS.

I had to agree with him on how sad his life had been. Earl continued telling me about his failed relationships and how drugs seemed to numb the pain. He said he felt so guilty about his life and questioned whether AIDS was God's punishment.

I reminded him that it wasn't all his fault. People who were abused as children tend to fall into the pattern of abuse as adults. I suggested that some of his guilt was self-imposed. Not that he was a total victim, but that life is complicated. He didn't have to be so hard on himself.

"As for God," I said, "I want you to know that God doesn't punish people by giving them AIDS." I told him the story about the blind man who was brought to Jesus. "Who sinned, this man or his parents, that he was born blind?" the people wanted to know. Jesus answered, "Neither this man nor his parents are to blame. But God's power can be revealed in this man's healing." I explained what Jesus was saying, that sin and sickness are not necessarily linked up as cause and effect as everybody in that time believed.

"When a person has AIDS," I told Earl, "God comes very close and offers help in time of need. We are much harder on ourselves than God is. We think we don't deserve God's love, acceptance, and forgiveness. But God thinks we're worth it!"

"I'm not a religious person," admitted Earl. "Why would God want to help me now that I'm sick? I never asked him for anything in all my life, and now it's too late."

"*It's never too late*," I told Earl. "It's often the case that we find God late . . . at a point when we really need help.

Coming to God when you need him is a really good time to come to God!"

It seemed obvious to me that Earl was seeking the God who was seeking him. I offered to pray with him. He said okay. I prayed, asking for forgiveness, faith, and a new perspective for his sad life. I prayed for strength for Earl to face what was ahead. Most of all I prayed that God would draw near in love and presence. I was holding Earl's hand. He had tears in his eyes. I knew in my heart he was drinking from the well of forgiveness and would be one *who loved much*.

It was six months before I saw Earl again in the hospital. Remembering our earlier encounter, he was quick to tell me how often he had thought about the things we shared. Life was still hard and painful, but something was different. I discerned a greater depth of character and a changed heart.

Earl asked me how my church was doing. I replied that we lost our worship center in the earthquake, and that our emergency shelter was housing some of the displaced families who lost their homes in the quake.

He was visibly moved. "I don't like to see people suffering," he said. He reached for his wallet in the drawer beside his bed. He pulled out a $20 bill and gave it to me. "This is a donation for your church. I've been wondering how to make a contribution."

I asked Earl if he were sure he could manage to be so generous at this time (he had recently lost his disability insurance). He assured me he could manage, and I thanked him for his offering.

Earl's spontaneous gesture reminded me of the sinful woman who poured perfume on Jesus' feet as an expression of her love. Her grateful heart revealed that God was at work in her life, that she was indeed forgiven. Earl's simple offering was no less revealing of a heart enlarged by the Savior's love for one who had been forgiven much.

As I prepared to leave, his partner, Jim, arrived in the

room. Suddenly, I was reminded that Earl was gay and that my church tends to put restrictions on God's grace.

Earl received forgiveness on God's terms, not the church's. He came to Christ not by renouncing his homosexuality, but by simply recognizing the emptiness of his life without God. His repentance was a matter of the heart; his faith was expressed in his generosity and gratitude. His conversion did not fit the contemporary evangelical norm, but is closer to the Gospel narratives in revealing the work of God below the surface.

Do we dare to believe that God can love and accept a gay man with AIDS and his partner just as they are? Can we believe that God forgives sinners simply by looking upon their broken lives and hearts, and rewards their openness to love with the gift of grace and forgiveness? Can we believe that God, as our loving parent, will gently and patiently raise and reconcile those created in God's image? In God's time, in God's way, and on God's terms, salvation is accomplished.

Though the church may put restrictions on grace, AIDS ministry requires us to go back to the basics of the gospel of Jesus: The Messiah is here, and the Kingdom is at hand. God loves us whether or not we return that love. We are understood and accepted even before we repent. Forgiveness is offered before we receive it as a gift. God never condemns. We only condemn ourselves by our refusal to love and be loved. God is present through *love, acceptance, and forgiveness*.

When we see people open their hearts and react to God's love in their lives, whether or not they fit the prescription for salvation, we recognize the presence of God at work to forgive and heal.

CHAPTER THREE

When AIDS Comes to Church

"If we are the Church, then I may come to you as I would Christ . . . just as I am . . . knowing that you will understand my tears, my anger, my sin, believing that somehow Christ will see me with your eyes, touch me with your hands, heal me with your love."

"OUR CHURCH HAS AIDS" was a shocking slogan to me when I first heard it used in a local Episcopal parish in San Francisco. I remember my immediate, visceral response: "Well, maybe your church has AIDS, but ours doesn't!" Then Joey, one of our Sunday school kids, was diagnosed with AIDS. And Lorie, a single woman in the congregation, became a foster parent of an infant with AIDS. Suddenly, AIDS was no longer a statistical or medical issue that we could debate in our safe circles of concern. No longer was AIDS an issue of us and them. AIDS was now our issue, for we had become *a church with AIDS!*

Golden Gate Community Church is not alone in its struggle to face the reality of AIDS. Increasing numbers of churches in all denominations are discovering that some of their own members have AIDS. What do you do when AIDS comes to church? More important, how do you become a church where people with AIDS are welcomed? Let us study and learn from the attitudes of one urban church.

First Church of the Open Door (not its actual name) is a growing metropolitan evangelical Protestant church. Its membership is largely middle class—business persons, teachers, nurses, students, and retired persons. The year was 1987, and they had heard a lot about AIDS. Because the composition and attitudes of this particular congregation may be typical of many evangelical congregations, the case can serve as an example of corporate assumptions to be overcome in order to undertake effective AIDS ministry. A church volunteer conducted a survey of the members of the congregation concerning their attitudes toward people with AIDS. There was reportedly considerable we-they language in their responses: "*They've* brought it upon *themselves!*" "*We* must hate the sin but love the *sinner.*" "*We* need to tell *them* God loves *them.*" "*They* need salvation, particularly as *they* approach death." "AIDS may be an opportunity for *them* to turn to God."

According to the writer who reported the results of the survey, three general perceptions are revealed in these comments: (1) AIDS and homosexuality are inextricably linked; (2) it makes a difference how AIDS was acquired—sexually or by blood transfusion; (3) a true Christian could not contract AIDS (except by a blood transfusion).[1]

Let us challenge these assumptions in the interest of dissolving the we-they distinction in AIDS ministry. Only then can First Church of the Open Door become a more sensitive and "AIDS-friendly" church.

"ONLY GAYS GET AIDS"

The first assumption—*AIDS and homosexuality are inextricably linked*—is based on how the disease first spread in North America. In 1981, rare forms of cancer and pneumonia were discovered affecting primarily the gay community and a handful of Haitians and hemophiliacs. Some in the medical community called the disease GRIDS—Gay-Related Immune Deficiency Syndrome—while the media often referred to it as "gay cancer."

---

[1] " 'Us' and 'Them' in a City Church" by Helena Kennedy, *AIDS and Compassion*, ed. Jim McPherson (Canberra, Australia: St. Mark's, 1988), pp. 65-67.

After the Human Immunodeficiency Virus (HIV) was discovered in 1984, the epidemic became widely known as AIDS. A few years and 100,000 cases later, the name was changed to HIV disease. But its original association with gay men stuck in the public's mind, even though the disease is believed to have originated in Africa among heterosexuals. In the 1990s, AIDS is spreading primarily in the heterosexual IV drug culture, among ethnic minorities, and in Third World countries where needle replacement is not a common medical practice. Still, the public perception is that AIDS and gay culture are nearly synonymous.

Since homosexuality remains a volatile social and religious issue, the stigmatization of AIDS patients is even more severe. The fact that AIDS is often a sexually transmitted disease (STD) raises suspicions in people's minds about how "good moral people" could possibly catch it. Though unfortunate, it is not surprising that so many Christians avoid people with AIDS.

If we as the church could overcome our reluctance to deal with sexual issues, our abhorrence of the idea of homosexuality, and our fear of disease in general, then compassionate ministry to people with AIDS would be possible.

As increasing numbers of persons who are not gay contract AIDS, the persistent stereotypes and deep-seated assumptions about AIDS as a gay disease will disappear. My wife, Rebecca, and I have a friend named Lorie, who was mentioned earlier. In her courageous and compassionate nature, we see the embrace of God toward all God's children.

God Is Like a Loving Mother
by Rebecca Laird

My friend Lorie is a "baby mom," which means she is a foster mother for medically fragile infants. As one of her sponsors, I went to the hospital to meet Patrick, who will soon be the second baby to come into her home. Patrick is a baby with AIDS; his mother died of AIDS three months ago. His father is nowhere to be found. Patrick was admitted to the hospital at the age of nine months for failure to thrive. He weighed less than ten pounds and found eating of little interest. This little tyke has too many medical problems to list. Needless to say, he's fought hard every day of his short life. He rarely cries. Small whimpers and wide, distant eyes that tear up are the only signs that he is in need.

Patrick's room on the pediatric intensive care unit is filled with two large teddy bears, a red, blue, and yellow mobile, a bag full of new clothes along with multiple tubes, gadgets, gizmos, syringes and monitors—all evidence of the hospital's caring. Many of the hospital staff serve as Patrick's "cuddlers." A seeming army of them with open arms stops by to softly lift the tiny black-haired beauty out of his crib and coo to him and rock him for a brief while.

But there is a sadness about Patrick that makes everyone work doubly hard to evince a small smile or to bring a glimmering sparkle to his eyes. As one of his nurses coaxed him to open his bird-like mouth for yet one more dosage of horrible-tasting medicine by chanting over and over, "You are a champion, Patrick, such a courageous little champion," a lump rose in my throat.

In this world full of people who are idolized and emulated for living well and high and fast, I was reminded that it is really those who barely thrive, struggle to smile, and develop slowly who are really the heroes. Patrick has suffered more in eleven months than most of us will suffer in a much longer lifetime. And he keeps on trying, keeps on watching person after person come and go from his room not knowing who is his family—or who will take him home.

In a week or two Lorie will bring Patrick home to her apartment where he will live until he dies. She, a single mother already dedicated to one fragile foster son, has chosen to love this doe-eyed little creature for as many days as he is given on this planet. Without a miracle Patrick will not graduate from college or even from kindergarten. He may never play little league or understand what it means to ask Jesus into his heart, but he is infinitely important to the lives of many, many people and to God. There is something so tender about an orphaned, helpless child. He reminds us of our humanness, of our need for a home and someone to care for us when sadness is all that honestly can shine forth from our eyes. Patrick represents the vulnerable part of all of us. And Lorie represents how maternal and loving our God must be![2]

After living with Patrick for a month, Lorie presented her son for Christian baptism. It was my privilege to baptize Patrick on the weekend of his first birthday at Golden Gate Community Church.

As Lorie and Patrick, Lorie's parents and godmother, Patrick's sponsors and care-givers, all gathered around the altar, I introduced the sacrament of infant baptism. Aware that AIDS babies like Patrick typically do not live past two or three years, I reminded the congregation that this may be the only profession of faith in this child's life, and that the vows said on his behalf today are efficacious and constitute the inclusion of Patrick into the household of faith.

Rebecca, Patrick's sponsor, read from I Samuel 1:21-28 about the dedication of Samuel. I asked Lorie, "Can you say with Hannah, who presented Samuel to the priest: 'I give him to the Lord. For his whole life he will be given over to the Lord' ?"

"Yes."

Taking Patrick in my arms and lifting him to God, I offered a baptismal prayer:

We thank you, God, for the gift of life, for you have given us Patrick to love and cherish. We thank you,

---

[2] Originally printed in *Herald of Holiness*, October 1989, p. 9. Courtesy of the *Herald of Holiness*.

dear Father, for the water of baptism. By it we are raised to new life. And so, we come joyfully into your presence, baptizing Patrick in the Name of the Father, Son, and Holy Spirit.

While we do not know how long Patrick will live, we do know that he will not die alone. Lorie will have him in her arms, those helping her care for Patrick will be a phone call away. The BRIDGE for Kids (sponsored by Golden Gate Compassionate Ministries) and other AIDS service providers will offer their resources. And Lorie's community will continue to be an extended family to mother and child.

Gay men are not the only ones who contract AIDS. Mothers and fathers, sisters and brothers, and young children have been and are being infected. By now, most people in the United States know someone with AIDS. AIDS has come to church, and the church must respond.

"BUT HOW DID THEY GET IT?"

The second assumption made by the First Church of the Open Door was that in ministry *it makes a difference how a person caught AIDS.* How often in my own AIDS chaplaincy work I watch people wondering whether a certain patient is gay or a drug addict, and how he or she got the disease.

This attitude is not simply one of curiosity, it is based on the fallacy that those who acquire the disease "innocently" through a blood transfusion or a needle stick are morally superior to those who were infected through sexual relations or drug abuse.

The reasoning goes something like this: "AIDS victims are usually gay or drug addicts, thus sinful. The Bible says 'you reap what you sow.' Therefore God is punishing them for immoral behavior."

Even my own denomination's official periodical, the

Herald of Holiness, published an article in 1988 favorably quoting an "expert" who sees AIDS as a judgment of God, "not simply on homosexuals, but a judgment on our country."[3] A few months later, it was reported that "two Nazarene pastors were infected with the AIDS virus," which begs the question—why was God punishing them? The news story was quick to point out that the pastors were infected "through blood transfusions or unsanitary medical conditions," not sexual transmission.[4]

IS AIDS GOD'S JUDGMENT?

How can we interpret the reality that AIDS frequently affects those whose *life-style* puts them at high risk?

In the USA during the first decade of AIDS, the majority of cases were in the gay community. Those in the gay community who had anal intercourse with multiple sexual partners were at the highest risk of exposure to the virus. In the late 1980s and early 1990s, the majority of the new cases of infection were among users of intravenous drugs. Those who reuse dirty syringes and needles continue to face the highest risk. The remaining 2 percent of AIDS cases affect hemophiliacs, recipients of blood transfusions, children born to infected mothers, and heterosexual partners of AIDS carriers. Pediatric cases are now the fastest growing group at risk.

If AIDS sufferers are simply reaping what they have sown, then why don't all sinners have AIDS? If AIDS is a penalty for sin, why is God so selective in who gets punished? Why do gay males tend to get infected and not lesbian women? Why is AIDS spreading faster among ethnic minorities than among the white majority? Are

---

3 "Church Should Back Sensible AIDS Policy, Says Expert," *Herald of Holiness*, January 15, 1988. p. 33.
4 *Nazarene News*, May 13, 1988.

blacks and hispanics, who account for a disproportionately higher percentage of AIDS cases, any more sinful than the rest? And why do so many "innocent victims"—newborn infants, hemophiliacs, and health care workers—reap what they did not sow? Is God ultimately a capricious deity who dispenses penalties indiscriminately?

The "judgment-of-God" theory of AIDS raises more illogical questions than it answers. It is predicated on a primitive view of God as one who sends plague and pestilence on those who do evil. Such a view denies the essential loving and merciful character of the God revealed in Jesus Christ.

The problem with "judgment-of-God" theology—attributing sickness and disease directly to God's intention to punish—is that it gives false justification for God's people not to get involved with those who suffer. As one Christian layperson asked me upon discovering that I was involved in AIDS ministry, "Why are you trying to interfere with what God is doing in the world?"

Smoking, for example, has been medically linked to lung cancer. If you're tired and susceptible, and you go out into the cold damp air, you might catch the flu. If you stick a contaminated needle in your arm, you might get infected with HIV. Sin and carelessness account for a large percentage of sickness and disease. But only a theology that attributes evil to God asserts that God specifically *punishes* cigarette smokers with cancer or afflicts drug addicts and homosexuals with AIDS. AIDS is a disease, as is cancer and the common cold. There are natural outcomes, not divine afflictions, from exposure to germs and viruses. Any other theology negates the revelation of God's compassionate nature.

The truth is—whether or not we have AIDS—we all have sinned and missed the mark of God's intentions. We all have failed in ways that did or should result in disastrous consequences. None of us has a leg to stand on before a just and holy God. If God wanted to punish us in this life for our sins, we might all have AIDS. If . . . but thank God . . . when we stand before the pearly gates to heaven, "Lord, have mercy" is the only plea that will let us in.

The Tale of Three Sinners
by Susan Foley

Once there were three people living in a certain city. One was an urban minister. This man had been born into a Christian family and the message of Christ had taken deep root in him. He had chosen a Christian college, gotten a graduate degree in theology, and had come to the slums of the city seeking only to serve the poor and sick in the name of Christ. He founded a mission there, in the poorest and most desperate neighborhood; he fed the hungry, sheltered the homeless, and by his words and deeds many were converted to the love of Jesus Christ. The ministry grew. Others were attracted by the holiness of this one man, and eventually a large and famous ministry, which comforted and saved hundreds, came into being.

In the same city lived a woman of prayer. This woman gave her love to God in the silence of prayer from her earliest childhood. Coming to maturity, she spent hours each day in prayer, as well as raising her family in the fear of God. She and the minister were friends, helping and encouraging each other. It was not known to any on earth, not even the woman herself, but through her ministry of prayer hundreds of people were comforted and saved.

In the streets of the same city lived a drug addict. He, like many other addicts, had been born to a good home, but of his own choice had turned to sin early in his life. Experimenting with drugs as a teenager had quickly led him to selling drugs to younger children. When he became a man he often obtained the money he needed by theft and violence, preying on the helpless. He consorted freely with prostitutes of both sexes. His behavior was wholly lawless. Finally he found that he had contracted AIDS, whether from sexual excesses or from contaminated needles he did not know. As he died he whispered, in a voice too low for any to have heard him, "Lord, have mercy."

As it happened, the minister and the woman of prayer died at that same instant, and the three found themselves before a huge and beautiful door. When the minister knocked, the door swung slowly open, and they saw a luminous bearded figure, surrounded by a heavenly host. "Saint Peter," cried the woman. "We seek entrance into heaven!"

"Welcome to the heavenly kingdom," said Saint Peter. "However, before you are admitted, you are required to show at least two hundred merit points."

"Well," began the minister, "I founded a wonderful and effective mission to the homeless in my city. Hundreds of the dying were comforted, and hundreds of the lost were converted through my work."

"Very good!" said Saint Peter. "Five points."

"Since I was twenty I have attended church services every day," said the woman of prayer. "In addition, I spent two hours each day in prayer for the suffering and unfortunate."

"Very good!" said Saint Peter. "Five points."

"I sacrificed my own life and comfort to my ministry," said the minister. "I had no possessions. I devoted everything to the service of the poor."

"Good!" said Saint Peter. "Three points."

"I raised my children in the service of God," said the woman. "I served my family selflessly; my husband and my children were blessed in my care."

"Three points," said Saint Peter.

The drug addict hung his head in silence, having no good deeds to put forth. The minister and the woman continued for some time to list their accomplishments, but their total scores increased more and more slowly. When they each had about twelve points (and were running out of ideas) and the addict had, of course, none, the three looked at each other, the panic rising in all their hearts. Finally they all turned and cried together, "What will become of us? Lord, have mercy!"

Peter smiled. "Two hundred points," he said, and welcomed all three into heaven.

"REAL CHRISTIANS DON'T GET AIDS"

The third assumption of the First Church of the Open Door was that *no true Christian could contract AIDS.* This attitude, too, is based on a judgment of the morality and spiritual status of people with AIDS. The argument is reduced to this: God punishes horrendous sinners with AIDS. Real Christians do not sin horrendously. Therefore, real Christians don't get AIDS.

In reality, few people continue to think this way. Nonetheless, an honest perception deserves a reasonable response. The fallacy is threefold:

(1) "True Christians" may have been immoral and contracted AIDS before their religious conversion and consequent change of life-style. I recall an incident in 1984 when a gay man began attending an evangelical church until it was discovered that he had AIDS. He was asked to leave the church, and it took three weeks of prayer and a board action before the congregation voted to extend to him the hand of fellowship.

(2) "True Christians," through no fault of their own, may come into contact with the contaminated blood of a "sinner." I remember the anger of the parents of a child with AIDS who had blood transfusions at birth. They cursed the "homosexual who donated his AIDS-infected blood to the hospital blood bank." Believing the offender was gay and immoral was the only way they could understand how their son could have gotten a "gay disease."

(3) "True Christians," being human, may in fact contract AIDS just like any other disease. AIDS spreads in specific ways regardless of the sexual orientation or spiritual condition of the transmitter or receiver. Rabbi Harold Kushner explains in his best-selling book *When Bad Things Happen to Good People* that we must not blame God or the victim but recognize that tragedy and suffering are an indiscriminate part of human life.

The assumption some churches make that AIDS is a disease that affects "them" but not "us" is rapidly changing. As increasing numbers of Christians with AIDS come to church or make themselves known in church, AIDS becomes our issue.

AIDS Is Everyone's Issue

The response called for is a compassion that breaks down the barrier of "us" and "them," that commits to inclusivity within the Body of Christ, and treats people with AIDS with equal concern and care regardless of how they were infected. Such compassion must stem from an awareness that *anyone* potentially could get AIDS; "innocent" or "guilty," people who get sick need care.

When people in the church ask me, "What can our church do to help people with AIDS?" I respond: *Open your front doors and become an "AIDS-friendly" church.* Profile church members as AIDS-sensitive people of God, and include persons from high risk groups—including homosexuals, substance abusers, and ethnic minorities—in your church, and you will be doing your part in responding to the AIDS crisis.

A Church with an Open Door

Terrance, who lives in the Haight-Ashbury neighborhood of San Francisco, often walked passed 1525 Waller Street on his way home. On this particular afternoon, he stopped and stared at the sign identifying the building as Hamilton United Methodist Church. He saw that, unlike many other churches, the front door was open, and he felt the impulse to walk inside.

"I'd like to talk to the minister," Terrance said to the receptionist, who was accustomed to seeing strangers come through the door.

After finding out that Terrance was not there for food, shelter, or social services, the receptionist said, "I'll see if one of our ministers is available."

The minister made himself available and invited Terrance into his office. They talked for about a half hour. Terrance apparently had AIDS and had just gotten out of the hospital where he had nearly died. Since that frightening experience, he had started praying and seeking God. "I've done a lot of talking, but God hasn't talked back," he told the young minister.

The minister listened.

"I've been thinking of getting involved in a church again, very, very slowly," Terrance explained. "I saw that this was a Methodist church and my folks were Methodists. I haven't been part of any organized religion for nearly twenty years. But I noticed that the door of the church was open, and something inside me said to wander in."

"Maybe God is trying to tell you something," said the minister.

"Well, maybe."

Terrance told his story and the minister listened. In the course of the conversation, the minister explained the church's open-door policy: "Hamilton is a 'reconciling congregation.' That means that everyone is welcome, including gays and lesbians and people with AIDS."

"When you say gay people are welcome, are you trying to change their orientation?" asked Terrance, noticeably concerned. "Because if you're into that, I don't want to have anything to do with you! Even though I'm not very sexual these days, I know who I am."

"No, the 'reconciling congregation movement' affirms the dignity, worth, and full participation of *all* God's people, including gays and lesbians, in the life of the church.

"Here at Hamilton we believe in the radical nature of grace—that we are unconditionally loved and accepted by God. Only when we deeply know and feel this truth can we begin to deal with our lives. The good news is that God loves and accepts us as we are with our commitment to become all that God intends us to be!

"We don't have to change before God will love and accept us. We come into relationship with God just as we are and find ourselves progressively being changed into God's image. Whether we are black or white, rich or poor, young or old, gay or straight—there is a place in God's kingdom and in Christ's Church for each of us. No one is left out!"

Terrance listened intently to the minister and asked questions. In the process, he was reminded of long-forgotten aspects of his own religious background. Terrance seemed hopeful and said he would be back.

"If we are the church," says musician Ken Medema, "then I may come to you as I would to Christ . . . just as I am . . . knowing that you will understand my tears, my anger, my sin, believing that somehow Christ will see me with your eyes, touch me with your hands, heal me with your love."

In order to counter the assumption that "true Christians don't get AIDS" and be healing instruments for those who do have the disease, we must recognize the true nature and composition of the Church. *We are the Body of Christ, and we have AIDS.*

CHAPTER FOUR

We Are the Church and We Have AIDS

"I wish my father would stop trying to account for me in his theology. He doesn't have to change anything about his beliefs. I just want him to be with me when I die."

After twenty reckless years of running away from God and the church that ordained him, the Reverend Tom Stibling reclaimed his Christian faith and desired to minister once again. AIDS brought him back to God, and the Lamb's Church in New York City embraced his gifts and calling.

Pastor David Best invited Tom to teach a Bible study, preach, serve communion on Sundays, and live as a minister in residence at the Lamb's. A group of Christian leaders surrounded Tom and encouraged him in his desire to start an AIDS ministry. Unfortunately, Tom died before his vision for an AIDS home could be realized. But he left behind the legacy and witness that God can use a minister with AIDS to embody the radical grace of God.

Most churches have members who have been touched by AIDS. Some are outspoken, and others are afraid to let anyone know for fear that they will suffer further embarrassment or rejection. How can your church become an "AIDS-friendly" church? How can your church become willing to put into practice the truth that God's love excludes no one?

To answer these questions, we will study: (1) What is the

Church? (2) Who can worship? (3) Who belongs to the body? and (4) Paul's teaching on "One body, many parts." In so doing, we will apply the *doctrine of church* to people with AIDS, to homosexuals, and to other outcasts who are seeking to know and serve God.

WHAT IS THE CHURCH?

What do we mean when we use the word *church?* A house of worship? A bureaucratic institution? A local congregation of believers? An invisible communion of past, present, and future sinners becoming saints?

Most denominations have a carefully worded and official doctrine of the church expressing their belief about what Jesus meant when he said to Peter, "on this rock I will build my church" (Matt. 16:18).

The Wesleyan tradition, for example, understands the church as *both* a visible institution of organized congregations and an invisible, universal body of redeemed persons who may or may not attend a particular denomination. Any person who confesses Jesus Christ as Savior is part of the "One, holy, catholic and apostolic church."

Real differences exist between people of faith, but our spirituality in Christ unites all believers, in all places and times.

To the church, then, belong all kinds of people: converted Jews and Gentiles, people of all races, men and women, rich and poor, young and old.

The question is, can we apply this inclusive doctrine of the church to sexual orientation? To health status? To addictive behaviors? To cultural life-styles? If the answer is yes, then we have raised the issues of *how* to incorporate homosexuals, hemophiliacs, drug users, ethnic minorities, and other individuals at high risk for AIDS.

WHO CAN WORSHIP?

Jesus addressed an issue that divided Jews and Samaritans in first-century Palestine. "Our fathers worshiped on this mountain," said the Samaritan woman at the well, "but you Jews claim that the place where we must worship is in Jerusalem."

The Jews insisted on Temple worship in Jerusalem while the Samaritans established a provisional place of worship on Mount Gerizim in Samaria. Jesus cut through the peripheral issue of *where* to worship God by saying in effect, geography doesn't matter. True worshipers "will worship God in spirit and in truth" (John 4).

Recall for a moment the fact that the Samaritan woman at the well had five previous husbands and she was not married to the man she was currently living with. Jesus did not cite her life-style as an issue disqualifying her from rightful worship. Nor did he condemn her. Rather he invited her to worship God in spirit and truth, whether in Jerusalem or Samaria (John 4:20-24).

If we exclude people "living in sin" from worship and fellowship in the church, we are as guilty as first-century Jews who excluded Samaritans, lepers, eunuchs, and other certifiable "sinners" from the Temple. When we risk inclusiveness in worship, we open the door to those who desperately need health and salvation in Jesus Christ. The church then becomes a safe haven where real people, dealing with deep personal issues, are made whole.

Author and evangelical minister Jerry Cook, former pastor of the East Hill Church in Gresham, Oregon, discovered the secret of effective ministry among outcast groups, including divorced persons, youth hooked on drugs, recovering alcoholics, and fallen Christian leaders. "Love, acceptance, and forgiveness—those three things are absolutely essential to any ministry that will consistently bring people to maturity and wholeness."[1]

His thesis was readical in its implications for AIDS ministry.

People need to be saved, healed, and brought to maturity and wholeness in Christ *within the community of faith* rather than outside the church, Jerry Cook argues. Before a person in need will feel safe enough to commit to a process of becoming whole, certain promises should be made by the community of faith. Otherwise, they will not take the risk of being open and honest about what they are struggling with—be it drugs, alcohol, sexual orientation, low self-esteem, materialism, or despair.

The minimal guarantee the church should make to people coping with real-life situations is that they will be *loved*—unconditionally—no matter what. We must say to people, "God loves you, and I love you, just the way you are, under every conceivable circumstance. There's nothing you have done or could ever do that would make God or this community stop loving you! Even if we cannot support some of your choices and actions, we still love you as a person." Who could resist a gospel like that?

Second, the church should *accept* people without reservation, risking "guilt by association" just as Jesus did. Accept *anyone* who has a desire to know God into the fellowship of the church, regardless of how "sinful" or socially unacceptable we think a person is. Yes, a biblical case can be made that candidates for church leadership must meet the highest spiritual qualifications (I Tim. 3). And yes, sometimes "tough love" and accountability are called for but the only qualification for drawing near to God in

---

[1]Jerry Cook and Stanley C. Baldwin, *Love, Acceptance and Forgiveness* (Ventura, Calif.: Regal Books, 1979), p. 11.

worship and fellowship is belief that God exists and rewards those who diligently seek truth (Heb. 11:6).

The way Cheers, the local bar in the popular television series by that name, profiles itself is noteworthy. Cheers is a familiar place "where everybody knows your name." It is a *safe* place where everybody knows your faults and troubles. It's a *friendly* place of warm acceptance where one is encouraged to deal with life's problems with humor and support. What a paradoxical picture of three aspects of the perfect church!

Why is the local bar so often perceived as a familiar, safe, and friendly place, and the church as one of the most threatening places to be oneself? If our secrets are safe with God, why can't they be safe with each other in the church?

Human beings require love and acceptance in order to survive in the world. We simply can't live long in hiding or with rejection. Psychologists say that unless a person feels unconditionally loved and accepted by at least one other person, he or she cannot develop into a fully functioning and whole person. When we love and accept people the way they are—by including them in the life of the church—people will open up and find healing.

But will our acceptance of persons be interpreted as license for objectionable life-styles? Perhaps some will misunderstand our motives, but usually the person being accepted will understand. By loving and accepting a son or daughter whose values differ from theirs, do parents confuse their child about where they stand? If the parents model certain values, children know what their parents believe and what behaviors they would approve or disapprove. *True acceptance—defined as believing in a person's worth, dignity, and potential—is received as emotional support, not moral sanction.*

The third attitude a church should take toward those it

seeks to reach is *forgiveness*. No matter what a person has done, regardless of how miserably a person has failed, despite how blatantly a person has sinned—forgiveness is offered in Jesus Christ!

To forgive someone is to release that person from your personal judgment. It doesn't mean you agree with what a person has said or done. It doesn't mean that the forgiven person should not make amends. It simply means that you will not act as judge, no guilty verdict will come from your lips, and you will not play God.

The Apostle Paul reminds Christians to be "kind and compassionate to one another, forgiving each other, just as Christ forgave you" (Eph. 4:32). Since God alone is the judge (Rom. 12:19), we don't have to be.

The "judge not" commandment of Jesus (Luke 6:37) applies not only to personal sin, but to a person's spiritual status before God. We are not to judge whether a person's heart is right with God. We see only what is external— actions, professed beliefs, appearances—"but the Lord looks upon the heart" (I Sam. 16:7).

There is a difference between spiritual discernment and personal judgment. Concerning false prophets, Jesus tells us that "by their fruit you will recognize them," and upon recognizing them beware (Matt. 7:15-20). But he does not tell us that if we fail to see any fruit in a person's life, then we can judge, exclude, or condemn. God alone knows who truly worships in spirit and in truth. As my childhood pastor taught me, "discernment is for our protection, not for our judgment."

Applying this truth to people with AIDS is essential. If people are promised love, acceptance, and forgiveness through the common life of the church, God will save and heal. If people with AIDS are rejected because of fear or intolerance, the church will be held accountable.

What am I suggesting here? That we open the doors of our

churches to include persons with AIDS and other social out-casts in our worship? That we offer Christian fellowship to anyone who desires to join us? That we love and accept "sinners" without first insisting they "change their wicked ways?" That we forgive them before they ask and release them from our personal judgment? That we leave to God the essential matters of conviction of sin and the need for transformation?

Yes! This is exactly what I am advocating. Where else but in church—where worship inspires us to believe, where the Word of God is rightly proclaimed, where small groups of accountability and support are provided to help us work out our salvation—can we find forgiveness and healing? Where else but in Christian community can we find support to recover from our addictions, overcome our judgmentalism and rejection, and gain strength to carry on? If the church cannot welcome "sinners," where else are we to turn? If not the Christian church, God will raise up alternative communities of hope and reconciliation.

Before his fall from grace TV evangelist Jimmy Swaggart said that he would not give "two cents for a church full of sinners." After his fall he claimed to be a sinner himself. What would happen in churches today if congregations saw themselves not as clubs for the righteous but as recovery centers for those who are loved, accepted, and forgiven by God? If the church is meant for "sinners" becoming "saints," then we're all in this together; distinctions do not apply. *All that matters is that we recognize the Spirit of God at work in one another.*

An old Hasidic tale punctuates this truth: A rabbi asked his students, "How can we determine the hour of dawn, when the night ends and the day begins?"

One of his students suggested, "When from a distance you can distinguish between a dog and a sheep."

"No," was the answer from the rabbi.

"Is it when one can distinguish between a fig tree and a grape vine?" asked a second student.

"No," the rabbi said.

"Please tell us the answer, then," said the students.

"It is," said the wise teacher, "when you can look into the face of human beings and you have enough light [in you] to recognize them as your brothers and sisters. Until then it is night and darkness is still with us."

WHO BELONGS TO THE BODY?

After resolving the issue of "who can worship?" another doctrinal issue surfaces: "Are *they* really part of the Body of Christ?"

The issue of "separating the sheep from the goats" is not new. There was considerable turmoil and controversy in the early church over whether Gentiles could be Christians. After all, Jesus came as the Messiah of Israel. How could a Gentile be Christian without first becoming a Jew?

Since Christianity originated as a Jewish sect called "the Way," it seemed reasonable to expect converts to be circumcised, observe the Torah, and accept Jesus as the Messiah. The book of Acts details the struggle over whether uncircumcised Gentiles were eligible for membership in the Body of Christ.

Paul, the self-proclaimed "Apostle to the Gentiles," argued in favor of accepting Gentile believers into the church without requiring them to obey Jewish obligations. The official church leaders initially were against lowering the standards. It took the council of Jerusalem to finally work out a compromise resolution recognizing Gentile converts as Christians as long as they subscribed to a minimal number of rules and regulations (Acts 15).

As far as Paul was concerned, church rules were open to interpretation and subject to change (as both New Testament documents and church history reveal). He continued to argue for the full participation of Gentile believers in the church without the Jewish "yoke of bondage" (Gal. 5).

Similarly, the ancient church in the book of Acts struggled with and eventually resolved the ecclesiastical issues of whether or not God wanted Samaritans in the church or whether an Ethiopian eunuch could be saved (Acts 8).

It was Peter who in a vision understood the will of God regarding the inclusion of non-Jewish believers in the church of Jesus Christ: "You are well aware that it is against our law for a Jew to associate with a Gentile or visit him. But God has shown me that I should not call any man impure or unclean" (Acts 10:27).

The truth is radically clear: All who evidence the spirit of Jesus are part of the community of faith, regardless of race, gender, economic status, or social stigmatization. As Paul was first to teach, "There is neither Jew nor Greek, slave nor free, male nor female, for you are all one in Christ Jesus" (Gal. 3:28).

Is there an application here for homosexual Christians, for Christians with AIDS, and for others who identify with the Body of Christ but feel rejected? As we might say today, "There is neither male nor female, black nor white, rich nor poor, gay nor straight, ill nor healthy, for we are all one in Christ Jesus."

Born Again But Still Gay
by Tom Cahill

I do not call myself a "gay Christian." I am a self-identified evangelical Christian who also happens to be gay. I was "born again" the night I graduated from high school in 1962, the same year I admitted to myself that I was homosexual.

With a call to preach, I enrolled at a Free Methodist school, Greenville College, in central Illinois. I joined the Ministerial Association and Missions Fellowship. I participated in a Christian literature crusade in Mexico City, and saw many won to Christ.

I probably would have become a minister had it not been for an intense, bitter, soul-wrenching battle for spiritual victory as I prayed for God to remove the homosexual desire from my life (even though I was not sexually active at the time). By the winter of 1965, I had lost the battle, turned to alcohol in rebellion, and was expelled from college.

I chose to immerse myself in the practice of homosexuality, eventually becoming so good at it that I no longer had to practice. I won't bore you with all the sordid details. Suffice to say, that for the next eighteen years of my life, I had one relationship after another, none lasting over five years. Between relationships, I was as promiscuous as I was capable of being. I spent many lonely nights drunk and depressed.

One year, I even tried heterosexual marriage, but I married for all the wrong reasons. The marriage was doomed to failure. I did learn that heterosexual relations did not cure my orientation.

I moved to San Francisco in 1979 at a time when the gay liberation movement was at its peak. I engaged in sexual freedom, liberty, and the pursuit of happiness with religious fervor. For gay men without moral restrictions, San Francisco was heaven on earth. Unknown at the time, a deadly enemy was lurking in the shadows—the Human Immunodeficiency Virus. None of us had any idea of the horror and tragedy that was being sown through frequent sexual activity. Due to my personal tastes, I never became a patron of bath houses, nor did I engage in recreational drugs. Yet, it is nothing short of miraculous that my HIV status remained negative.

By 1984, the AIDS epidemic had ravaged the gay community, and I was an emotional mess. Helplessly, I stood by and watched more than thirty-five of my friends and acquaintances succumb to AIDS. I became grief-stricken and despairing. When someone you have cared about for a number of years is dying in a bed of pain and agony, it matters little how the virus was acquired. What matters is that God draws near.

In the midst of the AIDS crisis, I was led back to faith in Jesus Christ, my Savior by an intense personal ministry of the Holy Spirit. It felt like I was being pursued by the "Hound of Heaven." I remember going to bed very troubled on the evening of July 14, 1984. A crisis was building inside me, a great conflict demanding resolution. I thought of the most ridiculous thing—praying. Though it felt strange, I prayed: "God, I don't know anymore if you even exist. But if you do, please reveal yourself to me."

A mental image formed in my mind of a great barrier, stretching as far as the eye could see, and constructed of huge granite blocks, carefully cut and set one upon the other. This barrier stood between me and God. I was saddened to think that if I were to come to God, it would take too long to tear down the barrier.

When I awoke the next morning, I was immediately aware that the barrier of the previous night had been torn down. I was completely captivated by the presence of God, who loved me just as I was. All the garbage my life consisted of for the past eighteen years was flushed away, and I felt once again washed in the blood of the Lamb.

Seven years have now passed since that great awakening. I have had time to reflect on my Christian life as a gay man. I have learned to take the words of Reinhold Niebuhr's "Serenity Prayer" to heart: God, grant me the serenity to change the things I can; to accept the things I cannot change; and the wisdom to know the difference.

Wisdom has shown me that one of the things I cannot change is my orientation. Nor has God "delivered" me or given me the gift of celibacy. Though my orientation may pose some problems for me, and may not be according to God's Perfect Plan and Intention, God's grace permits some degree of latitude as I seek to integrate my sexuality and spirituality. I am finally in a committed, monogamous relationship, for which I thank God.

While I know that my heterosexual brothers and sisters will not soon accept the validity of a gay person professing a saving faith, I am assured of my own salvation. The promises of Romans 8:35-39 are something no one can take away from me!

At nearly fifty years of age, I still feel called to preach. But I cannot return to the church of my youth. I love the Free Methodist Church, for it nurtured me in the faith and introduced me to Jesus Christ. But the church I love despises me, and it hurts too much to go back.

Instead, I am compelled to bring the good news of grace to the gay community which is shunned by heterosexuals. Despite the church's rejection, there has been a spiritual awakening in the gay community, largely due to the impact of AIDS on our lives. That spirituality has found expression in many ways and forms, including evangelical "born again" experience. I am sure there will be gay people in heaven as well as heterosexuals in hell.

As long as church doctrine maintains the view that all homosexuals are reprobates outside the realm of grace, there will be no understanding. Jesus held out his hand to all who would simply follow him. Can the church do any less?

With the challenge of Tom Cahill's testimony in mind, let us turn to the classic teaching on the nature of the body of Christ in Paul's first letter to the Corinthians.

"ONE BODY, MANY PARTS"

Paul in I Corinthians 12 defines the church as the component parts of an organism that confesses Jesus Christ as Lord. He then compares the church to a human body, and exhorts each member to understand him or herself as part of the greater whole. In his pivotal exhortation, Paul makes several points.

The body is a unit, though it is made up of many parts. The same is true with the Body of Christ—the church. We are many parts, but we are all baptized by one Spirit into one universal body without distinction or barriers that divide. This means we are not to distinguish those who have AIDS from those who do not have AIDS, but to think in terms of "our church has AIDS." We are not to draw distinctions between Christians in recovery from drugs and alcohol and those who do not deal with these particular issues, for we are all in recovery from sin. Nor are we to divide the body into two camps of "gay" or "straight," for we are all one body.

Because the body is composed of many parts, no part can say "because I am different, I do not belong to the body." If the foot, for example, should say, "because I am not a hand, I do not belong to the body," it would not for that reason cease to be part of the body. What if every part were the same? A body composed of feet? A body composed of hands? A body composed of eyes? Preposterous! All parts of a body are different and connected so that the body as a whole can function as a unit. In fact, God has arranged each and every part of the body just as they were intended to be. Therefore, in the church of Jesus Christ, there are many parts, but they form one Body.

This means that a person with AIDS is not to say, "because I am not a healthy member, I am not part of the Body." A homosexual member of the Body is not to say, "because I am not attracted to members of the opposite sex, I am not part of the Body." A black single welfare mother is not to say "because I am not white, married, and financially stable, I am not part of the Body." No. Together we are the Church—one Body with many parts.

Paul goes on to his main point: Can one part of the body say to another part of the body, "I have no need of you?" Can the eye say to the hand or the head to the feet, "I don't need you?" Of course not. It would be a denial of the interdependence of the Body of Christ.

This means that men cannot say to women in the church, "We have no need of you." The rich cannot say to the poor, "We have no need of you." The healthy cannot say to sick, "We have no need of you." The truth is, each part has need of others' gifts in order for the Body as a whole to function.

Because we need each other, those parts of the Body that we think are "less honorable" should be treated with "special honor," says Paul. Those parts of the Body that are "unpresentable" should be treated with special care and modesty, while the so-called "presentable" parts need no special treatment. To what is Paul referring?

As I reflect on this point, I can't help thinking of the called and gifted women in churches who must remain subservient because church doctrine or practice requires that only men be honored with leadership roles. I can't help thinking of people with AIDS who feel despised, dispensable, and unpresentable. Yet, if I believe in the nature of the church as described by Paul, each and every part of the Body is gifted, valuable, and essential for the whole.

Paul goes a step further with the analogy. One might think that the "honorable" parts, like the head pastor, should receive the most honor. But God reverses the expectation and elevates the least honorable to the highest place. In Christian community, the first shall be last and the last first. The humble will be exalted and the proud brought down. The poor are blessed while the rich are sent away empty. The greater honor should always go to that part that lacked it!

This means that the poor are entitled to mansions in the Kingdom. People with AIDS will have front-row seats at the Great Banquet at the end of the age. The first will be last and the last will be first. The proud will tumble while the humble will be exalted.

Authentic Christian community will reflect the order and priorities of the Kingdom. God delights in reversing social status and turning the structures in society and in the church upside down (see Luke 6:20-36). God's reason for doing so is for the sake of equity, "so that there shall be no division in the Body of Christ, but that its parts should have equal concern for each other."

Divisions happen when we make distinctions and distance ourselves from each other, assuming our differences translate into greater or lesser value. When one part of the Body thinks of itself as better than another, all that the "greater" part can show to the "lesser" is paternal pity, perpetuating the we-they distinction and resulting in divisiveness. But if there is "equal concern" for all parts of the Body, then equity and compassion can be demonstrated. No longer are "we" the strong, the healthy, and the righteous ones; and "they" the weak, the sick, and the sinful ones. Together, we are the Body of Christ.

The passage draws one final implication: "If one part of the body suffers, every part suffers with it, just as if one part is honored, every part rejoices with it" (v. 26). This doesn't happen in a divided body. But in a united Body, what happens to one affects the rest, for better or worse. When one part of the Body has AIDS, for example, the whole Body suffers. And when one part of the Body is healed, the whole Body can rejoice!

Paul concludes with the simple yet powerful reminder—"Now you are the Body of Christ, and each one of you is a part of it" (v. 27).

These scriptural implications clearly point to a doctrine of *inclusiveness*, even if other Bible verses appear to justify exclusion. All who confess Christ—regardless of individual differences in race, gender, socioeconomic status, psychological or medical diagnosis, or sexual orientation, drink from the one Spirit of God and are part of the Body of Christ universal.

The church is not exempt from the realities that impact our world. Drugs are an evil that has gripped not only society at large, but particularly the Christian home. Our own children are suffering from drug addiction. But we as parents and we as the church must not abandon them or exclude them from the transforming life of the church.

Homosexuality is a given reality not only in society but within the church. Some of our close Christian friends and family members are gay. We must love and accept them the way they are, and claim them as our own.

AIDS is a virus that has infected members of the Body of Christ. Personally, I have been in pastoral contact with scores of Christians who have AIDS. As family and friends, and as the Body of Christ, we must include them in our lives, welcome them into our churches, and believe that they have a place in the Kingdom of God.

Opposite Ends of the Spectrum

Frank is sixty years old and preparing to retire. A devout Christian, he has served the church all his life and expects to go to heaven when he dies.

Frank's son, Lane, is also a Christian. He attends a gay church and has AIDS. He neither hides nor flaunts his homosexuality. He dearly loves his father.

Father and son occasionally see each other, but there is

always unspoken tension in the air. Neither one understands or fully accepts the other. They need to better communicate the love they have for each other. AIDS is the tragic reminder that time is running out.

Frank firmly believes in the "dos" and "don'ts" of traditional morality. He wonders what he did wrong and why his son turned out to be gay. But there is no one he can talk to about this. Homosexuality and AIDS are embarrassing subjects in his town.

Lane would like to go home before he dies, but not until very close to the end. After twenty years of independence, he wants to do things his way.

"Lane, what do you need from your father?" I asked.

He replied simply, "I wish my father would stop trying to account for me in his theology. AIDS is not about him; it's about me, his son. He doesn't have to change anything about his beliefs. I wouldn't want him to. I just want him to want to be with me when I die."

Lane does not need a moral endorsement of his life-style from his father. He needs only love and acceptance. He needs his father to lay aside his moral concerns and simply be with his son. They can find unity and common ground, if they put aside their differences. They both have a place in the Body of Christ.

The doctrine of the church universal serves to remind us that together we are the Body of Christ. Some of us have AIDS, and some of us do not. Some of us are heterosexual, and some of us are not. Some of us are alcoholic, and some of us are not. Some of us have been forgiven much, and some of us have been forgiven little. But all of us are sinners loved by God and saved by grace. As the Body of Christ, we suffer and struggle with deep personal issues. As the Church of Jesus Christ, we challenge one another in love to become all that we were meant to be. And together, as the community of faith, we will find the healing touch of God.

CHAPTER FIVE

The Story of the BRIDGE

"I just live my live day by day, and keep praying my baby is healthy."

A man wishing to plant a tree in his yard was advised against the idea by his gardener. "The tree would take a hundred years to bear fruit," said the gardener.

"In that case," said the man, "we had better begin immediately."

Significant ministry grows from seeds in seasons and stages and takes considerable time to mature. The first stage is *responding to need and becoming AIDS-sensitive and aware.* The second stage is *forming a mission group.* Once a committed group has been in place for a year or so, the third stage can commence: *developing specific programs* targeted to particular needs. Finally, after three to five years of seasonal growth, a ministry begins to *bear the fruit* from seeds planted long ago.

Convinced that evangelical Christians need to embrace people with AIDS, Steve Worthington and I cofounded the BRIDGE: LIVING WITH AIDS. The work has barely begun, there has been considerable pain and struggle along the way, and the ministry has far to go before reaching its potential. Yet, in sharing in detail the story of the BRIDGE, I hope to point to a model-in-the-making, and witness to the truth that only as people work together in community can personal callings be fulfilled.

AIDS AWARENESS IN THE CHURCH

The way to begin is by *responding to need.* In 1983, the AIDS crisis had just begun, and I had not yet met a person with AIDS. In the fall, Malcolm's family contacted me. Malcolm had left the church twenty years before because he was gay, and his church did not know how to respond to him. He embraced the gay community of San Francisco and eventually contracted the AIDS virus, as did his partner.

I invited Malcolm to church, but he said his partner was quite ill. They didn't feel comfortable coming to services due to the unknown risk their presence might have been to others. (This was still early in the epidemic before the medical facts were known.) He preferred a counseling relationship, and we stayed in touch.

As he and his longtime companion struggled with the issues of living with AIDS, they both returned to their religious roots. The story of their acceptance by Malcolm's mother and her home church is beautifully told by Clarence Kinzler, a friend of Malcolm and the District Superintendent for the Northern California District of the Church of the Nazarene.

A Mother's Love
by Clarence Kinzler

Can a mother forget the baby at her breast and have no compassion on the child she has borne? Though she may forget, I will not forget you. See, I have engraved you on the palms of my hands. (Isa. 49:15)

Malcolm loved his mother, and she loved him. She raised him to be a sensitive and loving Christian in the church. Malcolm and I were friends in college. He played the piano with finesse. A few of us who sang formed a gospel quartet that traveled for the college. We were all very close and knew one another well. Yet, we didn't know at the time that Malcolm was gay.

I lost touch with Malcolm after graduation. I went to seminary, and he moved to California. Twenty years passed, and then I heard the news that Malcolm had AIDS.

His mother quickly flew to his side. It didn't matter that her son had a partner who also had AIDS. All that mattered was that Malcolm needed his mother's love.

I doubt if she understood the risks of AIDS or had a theology for homosexuality. She responded as any mother would, and cared for her son, and the one her son loved. Despite the unknown risks at the time (this was 1983) she became their care-giver.

Malcolm's partner was the first to succumb to the ravages of AIDS. She nursed him in their home until he died.

Malcolm did not want to live alone, so his mother took him back to her home where he could live out his days. Malcolm's final year of life was spent with joy in knowing he was accepted by family and friends. The church where he was raised invited him to use his gift and play the piano once again for services. He finally died in his mother's arms, at peace with God and with the church he loved.

Malcolm's funeral is one I will never forget. I will never be the same. AIDS is not other people's issue, but it is affecting our very own. We must respond.

I believe it was Malcolm's life and death that opened the door to AIDS ministry in my denomination. My district superintendent became responsive to the need and issued a mandate for Nazarene churches to get involved. "We can no longer deny the threat of AIDS or push it under the rug," the Reverend Kinzler told the District Assembly in his annual report on May 12, 1988. "The world is on fire with this ravaging disease. It's time to face our loving responsibility as the people of God. Just as Jesus moved toward the leper of his day and touched him, so also we must move toward those suffering with AIDS." In July of the same year, the denomination sponsored an AIDS conference in New York drawing medical professionals, social workers, care-givers, and students from across the country. The conference itself and the educational materials it produced were major breakthroughs in evangelical AIDS awareness.

Malcolm was not the only Nazarene with AIDS who desired to make peace with God and the church before he died. Others came into our lives and are to be remembered. We felt their pain. We shared a word of hope. We learned to journey with them through the darkness. They convinced us that God was calling our church to AIDS ministry.

In the fall of 1987, Joey Benko, a child with AIDS, and his family came to church and were "adopted" by our community and mission. We assisted them at critical points along the way in their battle with AIDS. Their situation became the rallying cry for action, calling forth a compassionate response not only from our church but from the whole city of San Francisco. (Joey's story, as told in *City Streets, City People* [Nashville: Abingdon Press, 1987] is updated here.)

Joey's Family

How do you tell a six-year-old he has AIDS?

We met Joey in the summer during a puppet show sponsored by our ministry at the public housing project where his family lived.

By that fall, Joey had developed respiratory distress. He was taken to the hospital and subjected to six weeks of extensive tests. On October 20, 1987, Joey was diagnosed with AIDS.

Church members met at the hospital to hold a vigil, anoint him with oil and pray for his healing. Just outside his room, we heard the young child's desperate screams and sobbing questions to the nurses: "Why are you hurting me? You're hurting my arm!" He had to be sedated in order for the nurses to change his intravenous line.

Once we were allowed into the room, Joey was only semi-conscious. Gathered around his bed, we sang and prayed and spoke lovingly to Joey, for whom the doctors had done all they could. "How could this happen to a six year old?" we asked the Lord in shocked silence.

The following week Joey was released from the hospital and sent back to public housing. His parents drew straws to determine who would tell him he had AIDS. Linda, his mother, drew a deep breath before she spoke:

"Joey, when you were born, the doctors had to give you more blood or you would have died. The blood you were given six years ago contained a disease called AIDS. Nobody knew it at the time, but now we do. AIDS is a disease that some people die from, but not always. All the church people are praying that God will heal you."

When his mother had finished explaining the situation to him, Joey cried.

Circumstances remained discouraging for the Benko family for several weeks. The family was assigned to a tenement apartment that the doctors considered medically unsafe. The neighborhood was high-crime, the housing project drug-infested, and the apartment unsuitable for a child fighting a life-threatening disease.

They suffered through a series of harassments, attempted break-ins, property damage, and physical violence. IV drug needles were found on their doorstep, windows were broken, their truck was set on fire, and the father was physically assaulted.

The frightened family needed to move, and Golden Gate Community did all it could to find a home, but no alternative was found. Other social services and AIDS advocacy agencies were contacted, but they too were unable to locate affordable housing.

We prayed for a clean, safe, and decent apartment where the family could focus on Joey's quality of life. We asked the Lord for a new home for Joey before Christmas Day. We created a ministry fund for "Joey's Home" and solicited sponsors.

Churches took offerings, individuals sent in donations, and social service agencies offered food, clothing, and furniture. *The San Francisco Chronicle* sent a reporter to interview the family, and ran Joey's story on December 23—"No Room in the Inn for a Child with AIDS"—and pledged to pay the first and last month's rent on any apartment they could afford to rent.

By New Year's Eve Larry and Linda's deepest prayer— "for Joey to have a home like it's supposed to be, like it's supposed to look and sound and feel"—was answered.

A small but safe and affordable one-bedroom apartment was located away from the drugs and crime. "And it's clean," said Linda with delight, "and with all the windows, it's very bright!"

The Benko family began the new year full of hope and the Lord's provisions. Joey eventually was able to return to school, and was put on regular doses of AZT—a drug treatment found to be effective in delaying the progression of the AIDS virus. Family and friends remain hopeful that Joey will live a longer than expected, relatively healthy, normal life.

Upon the publication of this book, Joey is celebrating his tenth birthday and his fourth year of living with AIDS. Although he has been hospitalized from time to time, his AZT treatment is working wonders in keeping him alive.

Since the day I met Joey, there has been a special bond between us. My wife, Rebecca, and I have enjoyed welcoming Joey to our home. He loves to play with our dog, Brewer, and to type letters on the computer. I'll never forget Joey's breakfast prayer one Sunday morning before church: "Lord, thank you for these precious years. Thank you for this food. And please help Brewer behave better. Amen." I love the company of this "old soul"—a child wise beyond his years—who has much to teach me about how to make the most of each and every day.

When Joey was first diagnosed with AIDS, some parents in the public school were opposed to having Joey in the same room with their kids. Naive about how the disease is transmitted, they didn't want their children to catch AIDS from Joey.

In contrast to the paranoia in school, parents in church embraced Joey and allowed their kids to play freely with him in Sunday school. In fact, one mother phoned me one Sunday to say, "I'm not sure I want to bring my child to church today. He has the flu, and I don't want him to infect Joey." What a difference of attitudes. The church had educated itself about AIDS and had become sensitive to those who had the disease.

Once a responsive community has become AIDS-sensitive and aware, forming a mission group may be the next stage in the development of an AIDS ministry.

FORMING A MISSION GROUP

It is helpful to avoid "reinventing the wheel" when starting a new ministry. The BRIDGE was built very slowly by following the guidelines set out in the *Handbook for Mission Groups* written by Gordon Cosby, pastor of the Church of the Saviour in Washington, D.C.—an urban church with dozens of successful programs serving the needs of the poor. The Reverend Cosby and his core community have spent nearly forty years in the city developing self-supporting ministries through mission groups.

A mission group, according to Cosby,

is a small group of people (five to twelve) conscious of the action of the Holy Spirit in their lives, enabling them to hear the call of God through Christ, to belong in love to one another, and offer the gift of their concrete life for the world's healing and unity. (p. 2)

Initially, a group gathers around a "visionary" or a small nucleus of persons. The visionaries are those who have heard a *call* for a specific ministry and have sounded that call in a variety of ways—in personal conversation, in leadership ability, or in prophetic witness. "The fire of God kindled within his or her own spirit inflames others" (p. 7).

If no one responds, the visionary must wait for the moment when others can share the vision. When two or three respond, they begin their "calling" together by "evoking one another's gifts, and praying for clarity in hearing God's will as to their mission" (p. 7).

The call may begin with one person sensing the still small voice (image, feeling) of God saying "feed my hungry," "shelter my homeless," or "comfort my people with AIDS." As others respond to the call, commitments are made to the group process. Servant leadership is essential here for the mission group to establish itself.

Then follows a season of praying for direction. Group members must educate themselves, work through the issues, and clarify their values. The entire group must write and agree to a mission statement, and become involved in direct ministry. In time, they must formalize their ministry structure.

In the case of the BRIDGE, after nearly two years as a mission group we launched a program to provide childcare in the homes of families living with AIDS. We also initiated an AIDS chaplaincy service for single adults with AIDS. Volunteers continued to meet as a mission group for emotional and spiritual support and to pray for persons with AIDS with whom we were in contact. Finally, after a change of leadership, the mission group disbanded. The BRIDGE continued its childcare program for families living with AIDS as an agency of Golden Gate Compassionate Ministries.

With this overview in mind, a breakdown of our three-year process of development from a mission group to a social service agency is given in the following seven steps:

Step One:

Sound the Call

Golden Gate Community has been involved in serving the needs of the poor and homeless since 1981. Steve Worthington, a charter member with a heart for reaching the gay community, was first to sound the call for AIDS ministry in the church. His call to start an AIDS hospice was based on his vision of countless thousands coming to know the Lord due to the outbreak of AIDS among gay people.

Soon there were others in the community who heard the call and made themselves available. We wanted to start a home for people with AIDS. We had a facility in mind (a vacated convent) and a project coordinator, but the dream was one whose time had not yet come. Instead, we volunteered at a nearby hospice center and provided services there on Sunday afternoons.

Two years passed before the call was sounded again for AIDS ministry. The occasion was San Francisco's first "Interfaith Conference on AIDS and ARC for Clergy and Care-givers" on March 21-22, 1987. Several members of our church participated with 800 others from Roman Catholic, mainstream Protestant, Jewish, and Buddhist traditions. To my knowledge, we were the only evangelicals present.

One of the conference conveners gave an impassioned

presentation on the need for the church to reach out with God's love. These words pierced my heart:

> The gay community seeking to care for their own responded first to the AIDS crisis. For this they deserve our highest affirmation. The medical community and mental health workers showed up second to the crisis. The doctors, nurses, social workers, and other professionals who cared enough to respond to what society called a "gay disease" deserve our next highest honor. Finally, the church arrived on the scene. Thank you for coming! Realize you're late, but we're glad you're here!

Motivated by the possibilities for ministry, I sounded the call to start an AIDS mission group in our home. Twelve people responded, including Steve Worthington, Bonnie Wong, and Rebecca Laird (all charter members of our church); Barry Brown, pastor of the church; Lorie Greer, one of the original nurses on the AIDS unit at San Francisco General Hospital; Muriel Beukelman, a sixty-two-year-old ministry intern with a heart of love; Jim Haynes, a mission board member who lost several close friends in the early days of the epidemic; and Holly Wake, a paralegal who was anxious for hands-on involvement with people with AIDS. There were three or four others who came to the initial group meetings but eventually dropped out, leaving nine original members.

We were empowered by a directive we heard at the AIDS conference: "Do not underestimate what God can do with a committed group of nine or ten."

Step Two:

Commit to the Process

After we had sounded the call and gathered the group, individuals were asked to make a specific and incremental commitment to the group process for ministry to emerge. In 1987 we initially committed to ten weeks of prayer and discussion. Then, we committed to stay together for a year as a mission group committed to AIDS ministry. Jack Pantaleo, director of the San Francisco AIDS Interfaith Network, met with us and recounted how he and a small committed group had prayed weekly for a year in the chapel of Grace Cathedral before the Episcopal Church responded to their request to hold a healing service there for persons with AIDS. After the success of the first service, other churches and denominations began sponsoring healing services.

We too were led to commit to a year of prayer in preparation for a healing ministry. I do not want to understate the essential nature of making a firm commitment to a call. Goethe in the late eighteenth century keenly observed the power of committed action:

> Until one is committed, there is hesitancy, the chance to draw back, always ineffectiveness. . . . The moment one definitely commits oneself . . . then providence moves too. All sorts of things occur to help one that would never otherwise have occurred. A whole stream of events issues from the decision, raising in one's favor all manner of unforeseen incidents and meetings and material assistance, which no [one] could have dreamed would have come his way. Whatever you can do, or dream you can, begin it. Boldness has genius, power and magic in it. Begin it now!

Step Three:

Work Through the Issues

Processing the implications of the call is an essential step to take *prior* to plunging into the programs of AIDS ministry. An insight developed that what God was doing *in* us was as important as what God wanted to do *through* us once we were ready.

During our year of prayer and discussion, we had the opportunity to educate ourselves about what others were doing in the city, and to work through several AIDS related issues: personal fears and risks, human sexuality, and death and dying.

We read all we could on the risks of AIDS and discussed our fears. We were fortunate to have known three nurses who had worked on the AIDS ward at San Francisco General Hospital, and called upon them to be educators. We watched videotapes and did our own research. Every week we would pass out resource articles for discussion and reference.

Still, after we were satisfied that the risk of catching the disease was minimal, there were emotional fears to overcome. What helped us work through the emotional issues was looking to the life of Mother Teresa. She started AIDS hospices in New York, Washington, D.C., and San Francisco. Mother Teresa offered these words to her volunteers:

> Maybe you are afraid like many have been afraid of leprosy. Many of your families are afraid. The doctors have explained all about AIDS to the Sisters. It is important to go into this work with confidence. There is now a big problem with suicide. Already two men have jumped from a tall building when they found out they had AIDS. If you are afraid, offer that fear to God. Do not force yourself. If you force yourself, you may be more preoccupied with the forcing than with the loving. What I tell the Sisters is, "If you get it, then you will die and go to heaven."[1]

---

[1] Quoted by Don McClanen in *The Ministry of Money Newsletter*, no. 11 (December 1985): 2.

For Mother Teresa, the issue is love and obedience to the call of God, not fear and risk. "God is speaking to us through this disease," Mother Teresa believes. Jesus Christ does not call us to a life and mission without risk. Rather, we are called to count the cost of discipleship and risk all for the kingdom.

The second and most difficult issue we sought to work through was our theology regarding gay persons with AIDS. We discussed whether homosexuality is genetic, acquired, imposed, or chosen. We debated whether homosexuals can change and become heterosexuals. We discussed monogamy as a moral option for homosexuals. We discussed whether there is a place in God's kingdom, and in the church, for the homosexual who does not have the gift of celibacy.[2]

We processed these tough questions as best we could through a careful and candid Bible study focused by the challenge of Andres Tapia in his article for *Christianity Today*:

> To avoid much pain and confusion, those who want to minister to persons with AIDS should resolve their theology and philosophy about homosexuality before starting.[3]

Although we did not achieve theological consensus, we did find spiritual unity. On the basis of Ephesians 2:8, we were prepared to accept anyone professing Jesus Christ as Savior as part of the Body of Christ, regardless of race, gender, social status, or sexual orientation.

We agreed that moral and ethical issues, such as sexuality, are best worked out in counseling sessions and accountability groups in the ongoing life of the church, and not made prerequisites of incorporation into the Body of Christ. We found evidence in Christ's life that he loved and

---

[2] See *City Streets, City People,* pp. 206-9 for details of our discussions.

[3] Andres Tapia, "How Churches Can Get Involved," *Christianity Today,* (August 7, 1987). p. 16.

42705

accepted people as they were and offered forgiveness to all who sought him.

For our AIDS ministry this meant that we were to welcome all persons without judgment, the way that Christ welcomed the outcasts of his day: "Come to me, all you who are weary and burdened, and I will give you rest" (Matt. 11:28).

The third issue we worked through together was our attitudes toward death and dying. We discussed both the terminal issues that AIDS patients face as well as our own experiences of facing death. We each told about the first person we knew who died, and about those we knew who had died of AIDS. Emotionally raw, yet spiritually empowered, we emerged with a depth of insight for AIDS ministry.

After a year of being together, one key member felt called to leave the group in order to focus on the needs of children with AIDS. This sudden loss resulted in a shift of group dynamics, hurt feelings, and misunderstandings. However, a "children with AIDS committee" was formed and the BRIDGE childcare program eventually emerged.

The remaining mission group members continued to meet weekly around the initial call to compassionate ministry among both single adults and families with AIDS, with a particular desire to see homosexuals reconciled with God and the church. Because the two groups were distinct in their callings, the mission group decided to go back to basics—to prayer and proven principles from the *Handbook for Mission Groups*. One of the principles is to develop a clear mission statement.

Step Four:

Write a Mission Statement

A mission statement is simply a concise statement of purpose that reflects the group's values, theology, and philosophy of ministry; and identifies what needs the ministry will address and what services it will provide. While it may not be necessary for a mission group to have complete theological agreement, members must have enough in common to work together in harmony toward the highest values.

Writing a concise mission statement is a challenge. If an AIDS mission group, for example, values renunciation of homosexual sin, clear-cut conversion, and prescriptions for salvation, that group will develop a mission statement emphasizing the importance of its members' discussing what the Bible says about homosexuality with AIDS patients they encounter. If, on the other hand, a mission group values emphasizing God's unconditional love and acceptance, that group will develop a mission statement that reflects these more relational values.

The mission group giving rise to the BRIDGE adopted the following mission statement in the spring of 1988:

> We are committed to a ministry of peace and reconciliation between persons with AIDS and the Christ who loves them, and homosexual persons and the Church that needs them.
>
> Toward this aim, we will pray for persons with AIDS, withhold moral judgment from those who suffer, listen to those who struggle with faith, open our hearts to those with gifts to share, adopt those who want us, encourage those whom God is drawing, and guide people toward a saving knowledge of Jesus Christ.
>
> Specifically, we are called to support those in our own church and mission family who live with the fear of AIDS, especially social service clients and children with AIDS. We will also extend ourselves in God's love to others outside our immediate community who by divine providence cross our path. (Adopted May 1988 through January 1990.)

It is obvious that we felt strongly about a compassionate, relational, non-judgmental approach to AIDS ministry. As the mission group's leader, I often found myself reminding both old and new members of the position we agreed to take: "We're not here to endorse or sanction anyone's life-style. Neither are we here to judge or condemn. We are here to love, accept, and serve people with AIDS, just as they are. We are here to witness to the compassion of Christ, who forgives and heals. We do not define ourselves as *pro-gay* or *anti-gay*! We are *anti-sin* and *pro-people*."

Sin, as we understood it from our Wesleyan theology, is not a moralistic or technical violation of God's absolute standards of perfection and intention. Sin is a relational and willful matter of the heart. Whatever violates my spiritual relationship with God or causes injury to myself to others, that is sin.

John Wesley defined sin as a "willful transgression of the known law of God." Father William, a trappist monk for thirty years, met with our group and offered a Catholic perspective: "Sin," he said, "is refusal to love and be loved."

Likewise, faith, as we understood it, is not a technical or moralistic matter. It, too, is a willful, relational response to God's initiative.

We found ourselves in agreement with Søren Kierkegaard, who states in *Sickness unto Death*, "The opposite of sin is not virtue, but faith" (p. 82). Faith is a fundamental attitude of the heart that is open to God, responsive to being spiritually led, and in personal relationship with God.

Since a person's relationship of faith is known only to God, it is simply not helpful to tell people how sinful we think they are. Instead, we are called to be instruments of peace that soften hearts and help people open up to God's great love! This is especially needed in AIDS ministry!

If a mission group can settle on shared values and a corporate theology and philosophy of ministry, then together they can move forward toward identifying specific needs and determining particular services to provide. If a mission group remains divided in purpose, as in the case of the BRIDGE, ministry will be delayed.

Step Five:

Nurture Gifts for Ministry

Gordon Cosby teaches that commitment to community effort is the basis for mission activity in the world. A mission group must come to value its corporate nature before an effective ministry can emerge. "This can be done only by discovering and calling forth the gifts of each group member," writes Cosby. "If even one or two members have not identified their gifts," he warns, "the problem of pride and envy will surface" (*Handbook for Mission Groups,* pp. 8, 9).

Multi-gifted persons who become visionaries, says Cosby, will face the temptation to satisfy their ego with individual enterprise rather than community spirit. Without a strong commitment to *community as the basis of mission,* even when this means unfulfilled personal expectations, effective ministry will not happen.

Mission group members tried to nurture each other's gifts for ministry. We discovered that not only was everyone in the group uniquely gifted, but each gift had a corresponding weakness. We found that we needed to work together if we were to benefit from each other's gifts. Such is the nature of the Body of Christ.

During this season of inward journey, we also initiated outward actions, such as "healing circles"—sessions for anointing and praying for the healing of persons with AIDS. It was to one of these healing circles that Daniel came for prayer by our group. His spirit was lifted by prayer with the laying-on of hands, and he came to value the power of God, even though he was not a Christian at the time. Daniel began to think of the mission group as his church.

Richard, a referral to our church, also found his way to our mission group and healing circle. He had prayed to receive Christ following his AIDS diagnosis, and was reunited with his family in Texas where he went to live for the rest of his life.

God showed us through Daniel and Richard that ministry follows commitment to community action where everyone's gifts are vital.

Step Six:

Create a Structure

Before we could formally create a ministry structure, the AIDS mission group and the children with AIDS committee had to be brought together. An agreement was reached to combine the two groups under one ministry umbrella called the BRIDGE.

A program developer was hired to get input from members of each group and design a five-year plan that incorporated the ministry concerns of all. The result was an ambitious plan in which everyone had a part.

When a mission group or a committee evolves to the point where a formal structure is needed, hard choices must be made. Should the ministry become separately incorporated or come under the auspices of a local church or mission? If it is to be incorporated, should its purpose be for religious or public benefit? Additionally, a magnitude of ownership, liability, and control issues, such as denominational affiliation and corporate sponsorship, must be resolved between all interested parties.

A church-sponsored AIDS ministry has both disadvantages and advantages. One disadvantage is that some social service agencies suspect your motives for ministry and may even accuse you of proselytizing AIDS patients and committing other acts of religious intrusion. Government funding is not as readily accessible as it is to public benefit agencies. Also, there is the risk that the sponsoring organization will wield church doctrine to influence and control policies and procedures that inappropriately limit the ministry's compassionate response.

The advantages of church sponsorship are the spiritual component it ensures and the service it inspires. If you can solve the matter of funding and resolve the issues of control, you can offer social services from a spiritual base rather than become one of many social service agencies devoid of spirituality.

The BRIDGE tried to structure itself both as a church-sponsored ministry and as a professional social service agency. It was incorporated as a nonprofit, public benefit subsidiary of Golden Gate Compassionate Ministries with a twofold focus: (1) to provide childcare for families living with AIDS, with a goal of operating a child development center for children with AIDS; and (2) to visit and spiritually support single adults with AIDS with a goal of creating a home for persons with AIDS.

Initial funding was secured from Nazarene Compassionate Ministries. With a formal structure and denominational sponsor in place, the BRIDGE was free to solicit wide support and seek volunteers from a variety of sources.

Step Seven:

Offer What Gifts You Have

After determining a structure and committing to a plan of action to achieve our goals, the BRIDGE began resourcing existing AIDS agencies in an attempt to test the waters and get our feet wet before plunging into the depths of program development. In so doing, we found out what other agencies were doing and what gifts we had to offer.

By the fall of 1988, a number of mission group members were involved in existing agencies. Steve Worthington was elected president and chair of the BRIDGE board and took on administrative duties. Lorie Greer left her job as a hospital nurse to become a foster mother for two medically fragile infants—a baby who was drug-dependent and Patrick, the baby born with AIDS.

Bonnie Wong learned her neighbor had AIDS and prepared to support him. Jim Haynes was trained as a volunteer with an agency that provides therapeutic touch to people with AIDS. Muriel Beukelman was trained in home care and became a home-care companion to two people with AIDS before they died. I became a hospital chaplain on the AIDS ward at San Francisco General Hospital.

By early 1989, several new members—all with personal callings to AIDS ministry—began working with the BRIDGE. For two full formative years, we had remained committed to meeting weekly. We were amazed to discover how many people with AIDS we were actually in contact with on a monthly basis (over one hundred) and the number of different AIDS agencies we were involved with as human resources (six). We were finally ready for a formal program of our own.

DEVELOPING A SPECIFIC PROGRAM

Although two initial ministries had been identified as possible programs of the BRIDGE, childcare for families with AIDS emerged as the top priority, and the single adults with AIDS ministry continued informally.

The BRIDGE for Kids serves as an example of how the

needs of a specific group can be met when a ministry focuses its efforts. At least ten steps are necessary in the process of program development and implementation:

Respite Childcare
Step One:
Target a Group at Risk

Linda Sallee headed the children with AIDS committee which targeted and researched the needs of pediatric AIDS cases in San Francisco. In the light of the staggering projections of pediatric AIDS cases, and with the encouragement of our sponsoring denomination, the needs of families living with AIDS became the focus of the BRIDGE.

Step Two:
Conduct a Needs Assessment

Linda and her committee spent three months collecting data related to children and infants with AIDS in the city of San Francisco by surveying AIDS service providers and medical professionals. They had three objectives: (1) to determine what resources were currently available for infants (birth to one year), children (one to twelve years) and AIDS-affected families; (2) to determine current need for services among this target group; and (3) to determine projected need for services by 1989, 1990, and 1991.

A total of 39 AIDS service providers were surveyed with 62 percent responding. Over half of the organizations that responded had received requests for services relating to infants and children with AIDS. The major needs identified by these agencies in order of priority were day care for children with AIDS (22.2 percent), therapy for AIDS-affected families (13.3 percent), hospice care, housing for family unit (11.1 percent), and support groups for parents and children with AIDS (6.6 percent).

Medical professionals warn that at least 20,000 children will become infected by 1991, and more than half of these youngsters will be orphans. In this same year, it is estimated that one out of ten pediatric hospital beds will be filled by a child with AIDS!

Step Three:

Define a Specific Service

Armed with hard statistics, the committee made a proposal to the BRIDGE. Knowing it was not equipped to operate a full scale AIDS daycare center, the committee proposed *respite* childcare services in the home—giving parents a break for a few hours each week. This program would entail community networking, identifying clients, home studies, case management, recruitment and training of volunteers, and coordination of services.

Step Four:

Find Funding and Management

The BRIDGE approved the program proposal and allocated enough funds to hire a program director, rent office space, and provide supervision. Golden Gate Community Church was the first to pledge monthly financial support to the childcare program. Individual contributors also committed themselves financially.

Step Five:

Hire Key Staff

Tere Brown, who had previous childcare, daycare and social work center experience, and who had served on the children with AIDS committee, was hired by the BRIDGE as program director on a half-time basis. Tere became responsible for coordinating clients and volunteers in the BRIDGE for Kids.

Step Six:

Develop Policies and Procedures

The basic policies guiding BRIDGE childcare services include: (a) *focusing on childcare* rather than on other issues that surface in the course of relationship to a family; (b) *limiting services to the client's home* rather than in any other facilities; (c) *confidentiality* of client's identity; (d) *monitoring health of volunteers* and protecting clients from contagious illness; (e) *home studies* of potential clients; and (f) *proper training and certification* of volunteers in CPR.

The procedures each volunteer is asked to follow include: (a) how to accept or decline a childcare assignment; (b) how to document the service provided; (c) under what circumstances to administer medications; and (d) what to do in case of an emergency.

Step Seven:

Network with Other Agencies

Tere contacted a number of AIDS agencies, explained what the BRIDGE was about, and offered childcare services to any AIDS-affected family the agency might refer. Trust of a church-sponsored AIDS agency by secular agencies had to be nurtured over time. It helped that the BRIDGE was one of the few AIDS agencies in the entire country offering childcare services to families living with AIDS.

Step Eight:

Recruit and Train Volunteers

It is relatively simple to recruit volunteers. Christians and non-Christians alike want to care for children with AIDS. It is more difficult to screen potential volunteers and select those who are competent and willing to be consistent in their commitment. During the first year of the program, a total of fifteen volunteers were recruited, trained, and certified to work with medically fragile children. Fingerprinting and TB testing were also required to comply with state regulations.

BRIDGE training is accomplished by medical professionals and involves basic AIDS education, children's CPR, attention to special medical needs of HIV-infected children and infants, and orientation to policy and procedures. Attendance at a weekly support group for volunteers is encouraged.

Step Nine:

Identify Clients

The goal to manage a client load of fifteen AIDS-affected families by the end of the first year was easily met. Some of the families contained an HIV-infected parent, others an HIV-infected child.

Step Ten:

Coordinate Services

The BRIDGE for Kids receives referrals from hospitals, the Department of Social Services, the AIDS Foundation, and other AIDS service providers. The BRIDGE recruits volunteers from other churches and organizations looking for a way to serve.

The program director spends her time doing studies of home environments and visiting families in AIDS shelters and hospitals, trying to determine the best course of action for offering childcare services. Once a family qualifies, they are linked to a volunteer who provides childcare in the home (or in the hospital) for up to four hours a week. The program director carries a telephone pager and is prepared to respond to her volunteers at any time. The story of Jana will suffice in profiling those the BRIDGE seeks to help.

Mother and Child in the Shadow of AIDS

When Jana, age twenty-five, gave birth to her son, she knew that she was infected with the AIDS virus and that her Jason might be infected as well. "It was stupid to get pregnant," she admits, "but now I'm so glad he's here. He's the only thing that has kept me going."

Jana considered abortion, but couldn't go through with it. Knowing that there was a 30 to 50 percent chance of her baby being healthy, she prayed the odds would run in her favor.

It is impossible for medical professionals to predict which babies born to infected mothers will develop AIDS and quickly die of the disease and which will be spared. Scientists understand and can prevent all routes of HIV transmission except that which passes the virus from mother to child.

"I just live my life day by day," says Jana, "and keep praying that my baby is healthy."

Jana has not had an easy life. A former drug user, she became homeless when she left her baby's violent and drug-addicted father. The $535 a month she managed to get from welfare barely paid for food, clothing, and her portion of the expensive medical bills. So like many desperate women, she concealed her infection as long as she could, and relied on the kindness of friends and strangers.

When Jana's son turned six months old, she contacted the BRIDGE for respite childcare. A home study was completed and volunteers assigned. She was grateful for a ministry that took a personal interest in her well-being as well as the health of her son.

The day that she was to find out the results of her son's HIV test was an ominous one. Jason, at least for the time being, tested HIV negative (exposed but not infected). The news brought deep joy to Jana, and yet, at the very next moment, there was profound sadness in not knowing how long she would be alive to care for the son she loves so much. For both mother and child, the challenge is to live one day at a time.

BEARING FRUIT

Ultimately, the BRIDGE hopes to open a child development center staffed by professionals and volunteers equipped to provide childcare outside the home. This will entail further funding and program development.

It could be said that our dream is too ambitious, too complicated, and too expensive to accomplish. To operate an AIDS daycare center will require much work, many resources, and an underlying faith and trust in God to provide.

In the face of doubt and impossibility, I am reminded of how Mother Teresa started her first orphanage in Calcutta. Mother Teresa was once an ordinary sister in a convent with a dream burning in her heart. Enthusiastically, she shared her vision of starting an orphanage with her superior.

"Well, how much money do you have?" asked the Mother Superior.

"I have two pennies!" replied Sister Teresa.

"Oh, you cannot start an orphanage with just two pennies," said the Mother Superior.

"No, but with two pennies and God I can start an orphanage," replied Sister Teresa. And she did!

The BRIDGE has an equally ambitious and impossible dream. Compared to the enormous cost of AIDS ministry, we have the equivalent of two pennies. And we, like Mother Teresa, have God!

"Nothing is impossible with God" Scripture reminds us. Even when it comes to meeting the needs of children like Joey, adults like Jana, and other precious people living with AIDS, nothing is impossible!

Compassionate ministry begins with the seeds of *responding* to needs the best you can, and becoming aware and sensitive to people with AIDS in the process. Formal ministry grows into being by *forming a mission group* and committing to the process of community effort. Ministry matures by *developing specific programs* focused on particular needs. Finally, what was planted can *bear fruit* when we count the cost and commit to its development, knowing God is Gardener in the field of ministry.

PART TWO

BECOME A CARE-GIVER

CHAPTER SIX

What to Do When You Don't Know What to Do: The Basics of Care-giving

"My father means well, but if he thinks I'm going to convert back to his religion just because I have AIDS, he's mistaken."

Every Tuesday morning sixty-seven-year-old Jessie Lee Ciupek drives thirty-eight miles from her home in Vallejo, California, to San Francisco General Hospital to visit AIDS patients. An American Baptist with a vital faith and deep compassion, Jessie Lee sees her work as an opportunity to show God's love. "People with AIDS often are leery of being visited by a church person," she says. "Some feel I've come to 'save' them or preach at them. There's a wall with many, but during a visit that wall can be broken down. I visit AIDS patients to let them know that not all Christians are out to cast the first stone."

A retired school teacher, mother of seven, and grandmother of twenty-two, Jessie Lee often finds herself as surrogate mother to patients who, for one reason or another, do not have their own mother close by. "Whether my role is mother or chaplain or just plain friend, I try to relate to the person, not the disease."

Jessie Lee's visits reveal the understanding and basic skills available to anyone willing to become a care-giver:

I knock before I go into a room. I call the patient by his or her name. I go in as an equal—not to be shocked, not to give advice, not to preach, not even to pray unless I sense we both have a mutual desire for prayer. I try to go in empty handed, without agenda, ready to enter into their pain—as much as they care to have me enter in. I listen, I care, I respond. Sometimes, a person asks for prayer. When they do, I always ask what he or she wants *us* to pray about. I hold the patient's hand and we pray together. I always try to follow the patient's lead, letting him or her determine what we talk about.

What do patients usually want to talk about? "The experience of being hospitalized, loss of job, strained relationships with family and friends, delayed payments from insurance companies, anger toward society, and facing death," says Jessie Lee.

She says the purpose of her visits is to offer a "ministry of presence," which restores power to patients. "They feel like they have lost control over their own lives. I want to help give back their power and dignity as persons in the image of God."

"Opal Gots AIDS"

Someone used a can of spray paint in the middle of the night to write a message on the front of Hamilton Church in San Francisco. There for all to see were the words: "OPAL GOTS AIDS."

Opal is in the hospital, confined to her bed. An IV line is hooked up to her arm. She must call for the nurse when she needs help. Her clothes have been stored in a box. She must wear a green hospital gown, which allows the medical staff easy access to her body.

Opal must eat to regain her health, whether or not she feels like it. The hospital is not known for gourmet cooking or fine dining. Although the food is edible, she has lost control over what and when she eats. She has lost control over her ability to bathe herself or go to the bathroom alone.

Her illness has robbed her of the simple dignity a healthy person takes for granted. To the hospital, her name is not as important as her number—what room and bed she is in, and what her chart says about her.

Nor does she have any privacy. Her health plan does not provide her with a private room, so she must share this loss of dignity with the person in the bed on the other side of the curtain. Almost anyone may walk in at any time. The doctor may come in to monitor her health. The nurse may come in to check on the equipment or change the sheets. The social worker may drop by to ask her to fill out forms. The person in charge of television rental may come by to collect for the rental. The food service attendant may come by to deliver or pick up her tray. A hospital chaplain or a friend may come by for a visit unannounced. These can be welcome interruptions or intrusions for Opal, depending on the sensitivity and skills of each visitor.

What Opal needs most is someone in her life who understands the experience of sequential loss, someone who will listen and offer her a *ministry of presence*.

Step by step we will examine the "ministry of presence," contrast it to the "ministry of absence," and commend the "ministry of practical support."

MINISTRY OF PRESENCE

"Being there is more important than *doing* anything," according to the Reverend Connie Hartquist, "and what you *hear* is more important than what you *say*." Connie is the Director of The Episcopal Chaplaincy at San Francisco General Hospital and Supervisor of the AIDS Ministry Training Program for Religious Professionals. After nearly two years of working under Connie's leadership at General Hospital, I am absolutely convinced of the ultimate value and effectiveness of a simple *ministry of presence*. The principles I pass on to you in this section find their source,

directly or indirectly, in her weekly training sessions and our supervisory relationship.

Suppose you know a person with AIDS and want to visit that person. Or suppose you have a calling to AIDS ministry and want to become a care-giver. How will the person know that you really care and want to be fully present in his or her experience? Hospital chaplains follow a seven-step process of visiting patients, which can be adopted by anyone who desires to become a care-giver.

Step One:

Prepare for the Visit

Why is it important to visit people with AIDS? Because when we visit and connect with them on a human level, the Spirit of God visits and connects with them on a far deeper level resulting in *empowerment*. It is a mystery of faith that in loving, human interaction and encounter, the door opens to divine interaction and encounter. Thus what we pray for and seek in every visit is the ministry of divine presence, which mediates, through our presence and through the relationship that develops, the healing, forgiving, sustaining, redeeming relationship with God incarnate through Jesus Christ.

To prepare spiritually for such a visit, I like to pray before I go, sensitizing myself to God's guidance, centering myself in the present moment. At San Francisco General Hospital there is a quiet prayer chapel on the second floor. If time allows, I go there and kneel before the altar. I pray for the Spirit to precede my visits and prepare the way, as well as to help me be fully present. If I'm on the run, I pray as I go, intentionally asking God to be with me when I visit and with the person I will see. Being conscious of the divine presence before a visit greatly enhances my consciousness of divine activity during and after a visit.

If you are visiting a person with AIDS at his or her home, it is best to call first to see if the person feels like seeing someone. Some days are better than others for home visits. If the time is inconvenient, suggest another day. If today is fine, be specific about what time you will visit and how long you can stay. Be sure to keep your word! There is nothing more disappointing for a person with AIDS, or anyone for that matter, than to gear up to see someone who does not show. When ministers don't keep their appointments, patients sometimes feel as if they are being let down, once again, by God and the church. Don't make promises you can't keep.

Before you enter the room of the person you are visiting, wash your hands. While limiting the risk of infecting the person with a germ, hand-washing has more than hygienic value. It has symbolic value of removing your own preoccupations and agenda for the visit. Prayerfully, you cleanse yourself of what you have in mind for the person in order to enter empty-handed. One thing that you want to wash away is religious agenda, however helpful and well-intentioned. Your need to pray with or religiously persuade a person may not be what the Spirit wants to do today. Offer God your free and empty hands during your visits.

Step Two:

Ask, "How Are You Doing?"

As you enter the room, knock first. (Very few visitors extend this courtesy.) Respect a person's time, space, privacy, and feelings of the moment. You are trying to restore a person's dignity and sense of control over his or her environment. Ask if you may come back later if this is not a good time to visit.

Identify yourself and the person you are visiting by

121

name. Chaplains use a simple entrance rite to get through the initial awkward moments: "Hello, Opal, my name is Michael, and I'm the chaplain on this unit. I just stopped by to see how you're *doing.*"

Don't ask, "How are you *feeling?*" That's the doctor's question. As care-givers, we want to ask about a person's experience of being ill, confined, powerless, and alone. I find a way to ask the same question—"How are you doing?"—three times and in three ways before giving up. After asking the first time, I might say the second time, "Opal, I know you've been in the hospital now for two weeks. How is it for you to be here?" If she is still not convinced that I'm really interested in how she is *doing,* I might say, "This may not be the best time for me to visit. Shall I come back at a more convenient time?" Usually, the response comes, "No please, this is a good time," at which point I ask if I can pull up a chair.

Sitting in a chair next to the bed is a clear indication that you care enough to listen, that you will stay long enough to find out how a person is really doing. And the person you are visiting will begin to open up. There usually is no one else in the health care system who has the time and interest to sit, really ask how the person is *doing,* and listen.

Step Three:

Attend to the Person

Care-giving is other-directed. It is important to pay attention to the needs of the person you are visiting rather than to what *you* need or want. We attend to the person as a child of God, not to the disease, the mood swings, or how the disease was acquired. By attending to the person, with a listening, loving presence, a connection is made and a window is opened to the Divine.

It often helps to sit close to a patient (but not so close as to violate personal space). Try resting your hand near the patient's hand. Be open to holding the patient's hand, but not too soon. Take your time in building trust and establishing rapport. Ask questions, not to get information, but to elicit feelings. Respond with your feelings. Elicit and enjoy whatever silence there may be. Silence is often an occasion for something deep inside to come to the surface. Don't talk too much. Smile a lot. Find nonverbal as well as verbal ways to convey warmth and care.

When you don't know what to say or ask, make observations. Notice what's in the room, including medical apparatus, flowers, pictures, cards, balloons. Comment on what you see in the person's environment. Ask about family and friends. Try to discern what's going on inside the person you are visiting, and then reflect back what you see. The person will correct you if your observation is wrong.

Adapt to distractions—television, visitors, other patients. Use distractions as opportunities to make other observations that let the patient know that you care.

Most important, embrace the present moment. Whether the moment is happy or sad, meaningful or flippant, there is in each moment of encounter the opportunity to share with another person whom God loves and for whom Christ died. There is sanctity in the present moment.

Step Four:
Build Trust

The only authentic way to build trust is to *be yourself, be accepting, be trustworthy,* and *be open.* Usually this process takes many years with acquaintances and friends. But in a hospital setting, with patients who are sick or dying, the process is abbreviated. Trust can be built in one or two visits.

Be yourself. Elizabeth O'Connor writes about *authenticity* in relationships in her book *Journey Inward, Journey Outward.* She says that when all is said and done, the greatest gift we have is sharing our real selves with one another. "We dip into our lives and offer what we find there" (p. vi).

Be accepting. Loving acceptance of others is the fruit of self-love, self-acceptance, and personal security. If you are secure about who you are, you will easily accept other human beings. If you are insecure about who you are and what you believe, you will tend to judge others. Love accepts, even though it may not agree!

Be trustworthy. Can you be trusted with another person's story of pain and rejection? How does your patient know you will not use the information against him or her? Before a person will trust you, you must show yourself to be trustworthy. This means keeping your word, visiting when you say you will, not betraying a confidence, not making promises you cannot keep, not trying to change difficult feelings.

Be open. All sorts of surprises await the care-giver who is open to new realities, new ways of being in the world, new ideas and belief systems. Being open does not mean you will agree with the other person. It means you are open to hear and consider what the other person feels, thinks, believes, and does with his or her life. Rigidity or judgmentalism in chaplaincy or care-giving is totally inappropriate.

Step Five:

Focus on Feelings

When we reflect on the conversation we are having with a patient, we become aware of two realities occurring simultaneously: *what is being said* and *what is being felt.* Since what is being felt is far more important than what is actually being said, the skilled care-giver focuses not on the content but on the feelings expressed in the encounter. Why is this?

The old, familiar, hymn by Fanny Crosby perhaps says it best:

> Down in the human heart, crushed by the tempter,
> Feelings lie buried that grace can restore.
> Touched by the loving heart, wakened by kindness,
> Chords that are broken will vibrate once more.
>
> Rescue the perishing; care for the dying.
> Jesus is merciful; Jesus will save.

Emotions are the wellspring of life, the primary source of thinking and behaving, arising from past experience in response to an immediate situation. To be conscious of our feelings is to be aware of our needs. To solicit others' feelings is to offer the support people need. Empowerment occurs when people are able to process their feelings in the compassionate and understanding presence of a care-giver.

The way we access emotions is to make astute observations, ask open-ended invitational questions, be comfortable with silence, and find a way to commune with another human being. We sit and listen to someone's story not because we are curious about the details of a person's life, or because we want a turn to tell our story, but because in truly listening to another, feelings surface that finally can be recognized and healed.

We focus on the emotional level of human experience by attending to both verbal and nonverbal cues of emotion. Verbal cues are solicited by asking invitational questions, like: "Tell me about your sister. Were you close growing up?"

Nonverbal cues are detected through making observations and reading between the lines: "I understand you to be saying that your parents haven't been able to visit you here; I'm wondering how much support you feel from them." Expressing your observations to a person elicits emotional responses and reveals what the person is feeling and what he or she is seeking. Nonverbal cues include body language, breathing rhythms, sighing, facial grimaces, eye expressions, hand clenching, silence, and tears. If someone has a tiny tear in their eye, for example, you could gently ask, "What's behind your tears?" Or "If your tears could talk, what would they say?" Be prepared to hear deep feelings needing to be expressed.

Step Six:

Offer Emotional Support

If you are truly attentive to the pain and emotion that a person is revealing in your presence, you will experience your own personal pain and feelings of helplessness. Your temptation will be to want to "fix it" for the person whom you now care deeply about. Remember that you are not the Messiah. There is nothing you can *do*, in terms of cures and rescue efforts. But there is something you can *be* and offer in terms of emotional support.

You can be present to the pain by sitting there and sharing without running away. This is something some families and friends find too difficult to do. But as a care-giver, you can "weep with those who weep" and "bear another's burden" for these moments you have together. If you can stand to do this, an emotional connection will be made, and God will be present in the pain of the moment, as well as after you and the patient have parted.

There are a few principles to remember when offering emotional support to someone with AIDS:

A. *Begin where the person is* on the journey of life and faith, not where you are or where you would prefer your patient to be.

B. *Don't compare* your patient's experience to your own. Stay out of the way. Your story is not what is important here. You are present to hear and help interpret the person's own experience.

C. *Accept the patient's reality*, whether or not it conforms to your own. Rather than agreeing or disagreeing with the patient, see what similarities you have with his or her point of view.

D. *Recognize your own limitations.* Don't try to solve problems. Realize that if you can be present to another's pain, it will be enough.

E. *Connect on the common level of humanity*, person to person. Meditate on the mystic notion that "nothing human is alien to me."

F. *Let persons know they are heard*, that you accept how they feel, that they are entitled to their feelings.

G. *Empathize, don't sympathize.* Attempt to understand and distinguish the patient's needs and your own. *Sympathy* is identification with another's pain and adding to it your own. *Empathy* is compassionate detachment, hearing what it is like to walk a mile in another's shoes but not stepping into the person's shoes. *Empathy* empowers a patient to rise above circumstances. *Sympathy* merely identifies with the pain and perpetuates it for both patient and care-giver.

Step Seven:

Offer Spiritual Support

At the risk of separating spiritual support from other kinds of supportive presence, a word of guidance is important. We do not offer spiritual support in order to convert people to our way of thinking about God. Any conversion to a particular expression of faith is secondary to the spiritual ministry of presence. The reason we offer spiritual support and comfort to persons with AIDS is precisely because we ourselves have been comforted and supported by the Spirit of God in time of need, as Scripture reminds us:

> Praise be the God and Father of our Lord Jesus Christ, the Father of compassion and the God of all comfort, who comforts us in all our troubles, so that we can comfort those in any trouble with the comfort we ourselves have received from God. (II Cor. 1:3-4)

When offering emotional and spiritual support, it is important to be invitational and responsive. Let the patient take the lead. If the person you are visiting wants to pray with you, he or she will ask, and you can pray together. Be open to verbalizing your prayers, but also realize that the patients may not want to pray right now, or may want *you* to pray for them later. Whether you pray with the person you are visiting or not, your visit itself is a prayer that reaches the heart of God.

If the person you are visiting knows you are a Christian and wants to know more about your religious views, the question will come up. Then you may share your understanding of Christ and the gospel. You may witness to God's love and faithfulness in your own life. Respond simply, briefly, and from the heart. Remember the person is ill and is not up for a sermon. But if they don't ask about your experience of God, don't impose your beliefs or testimony on them. To preach or moralize before an immobile audience is inappropriate. To confront what you think is sin or to try to convert another shows poor judgment.

Care-givers must be careful to respond appropriately with sensitivity to the person's needs. Christian care-givers are called to be gentle witnesses and reminders of God's love in the world. God's people are like *salt* and *light*. Salt is good only if it is sprinkled lightly. Light is effective when it simply shines. "In the same way," Jesus said, "let your light shine before men that they may see your good deeds and praise your Father in heaven" (Matt. 5:16).

In offering spiritual support to people with AIDS, it is best to keep in mind some principles of Scripture:

A. "Do to others as you would have them do to you" (Luke 6:31).
B. "Consider others better than yourselves" (Phil. 2:3).
C. Speak "the truth in love" (Eph. 4:15).
D. "Carry each other's burdens" (Gal. 6:2).
E. "Pray for each other that you may be healed" (James 5:16).

In the AIDS patient who is struggling with pain and abandonment, we see the suffering Christ. In the receptive patient, living more deeply with the advent of AIDS, we see the miracle of new birth. Even in the bitter, hostile, or depressed patient, coping with terminal illness, we recognize the essential self, created in the image of God. In visiting people with AIDS and offering spiritual support, we witness the invisible presence of God who dwells within.

From Hostility to Friendship

Paul's father called me from across the country in a state of panic. He had known for six months that his son had AIDS, and he had been in contact with him by phone. But he didn't know what to do in the light of Paul's anger and hostility toward his family and religion.

Paul was not even answering his phone. Where was he? Was he all right?

Members of the AIDS mission group were able to track him down in the hospital and found out that he had a brain tumor.

Knowing that I represented the church that he left in anger long ago, I prepared for the worse. What if he didn't want to see me? What if he asked me to leave? What if he was hostile? Should I tell him that I'm a Nazarene minister, or that his father called to ask that I check up on him? As I washed my hands I prayed: "Lord, prepare the way for a meaningful visit."

As I walked into the room, I said: "Hello Paul, my name is Michael, and I'm a chaplain. I just stopped by to see how you're doing."

Paul responded, "What brand of chaplain are you?" When I told him he became angry. "I don't know about this. Why have you come?"

I had decided to be totally honest and risk rejection. "Your father called me because he didn't know where you were. He was worried and asked me to try to find you."

"So, my father sent you? I don't know about this."

"Your father didn't know you were here in the hospital, and he sounds quite concerned. Shall I tell him how you're doing?"

"My father means well, but if he thinks I'm going to convert back to his religion just because I have AIDS, he's mistaken."

Paul invited me to sit down, and I became attentive to his feelings. I didn't try to defend the church or his family. I simply listened to his tirade on the church and his disappointment with his family, and I focused on his feelings. In the process, a level of trust was built between us, and we became friends.

In the course of our visit, we discussed his personal spirituality, as distinct from his family's brand of religion. He told me about his partner, who had died of AIDS. He told me how his pastor helped him reclaim a new faith in God. As Paul was revealing his heart, he started to cry. I sat there in silence, knowing that although he had abandoned the church of his youth, God had not abandoned him.

Our visit, which began with suspicion and hostility, ended with trust and spiritual support. When it was time to go, I told him that I would be leaving in a moment. Paul asked me to write down my name and phone number in case he needed to call. I was delighted to oblige. Finally, I stood up and said good-bye. Paul remained in my prayers and on my list of special people with whom to keep in contact.

MINISTRY OF ABSENCE

The *ministry of absence* is the recognition of the divine presence in our human absence. *Being there* is the gift we bring to care-giving. *Staying there* is God's part of the bargain. In our being there and leaving at the appropriate time, God draws close to the one in need and remains there long after we have departed.

How we complete a visit is as important as how we prepare for and initiate it. The key is in knowing when best to leave. The signals may come from the person or from within yourself. Either way, it is not helpful to stay past the time to go. You can no longer be fully present and attentive when you are preoccupied with the need to leave. There is also a limit to how much *ministry of presence* the patient can endure.

Once you decide it's time to leave, say that you will be leaving shortly. Genuinely express what the visit meant to you. Wish the patient well. Then wait for a minute before actually leaving. Often deeper issues will surface, and you may have to reassess the termination signals. Or the visit will end amiably, and the connection will enhance the next visit.

The "exit rite" for leaving the room is simple to learn. Stand up and gently touch the patient's hand or face. Sometimes a hug or kiss is appropriate. If you say you will pray for your friend, do it! If you say you will return tomorrow, keep your word! Better to simply say good-bye than to make promises you may not be able to keep.

After quietly leaving the room, again wash your hands. There is a cleansing ritual in the action. Commit your friend to God. Washing our hands helps us to leave in God's hands what we are unable to do, and to activate the *ministry of absence*.

After a visit, it is good to reflect on and pray for the person you just left. Instead of rushing off to the next thing on your schedule, find a comfortable spot to sit down and think about the quality of your visit. Making journal entries is a useful way to commit to memory those whom God has entrusted to your care. The way I like to end my day as a hospital chaplain is to make a journal entry about the patients I visited, then to go to the chapel and offer prayers for each one.

Washing our hands, reflecting on our visits, and trusting specific persons to God in prayer helps us embrace the *ministry of absence*. We can then rest in the knowledge that in our physical absence, the Holy Spirit of God continues to work behind the scene to save and heal.

MINISTRY OF PRACTICAL SUPPORT

Being there in the ministry of presence and *letting go* in the ministry of absence constitute the basics in AIDS caregiving. There are other, more practical ways of showing compassion. When a person is learning to live with terminal illness, even the smallest tasks become a burden. Assisting with cooking, house cleaning, grocery shopping, and transportation speaks louder than words. Help with housing issues, employment, and financial management is a living witness to God's love and your friendship.

People with AIDS may need someone to act as their "Power of Attorney" to help make medical and legal decisions about their health and estate. They need organized and trustworthy assistants to help them complete their unfinished business. Incontinent and bedridden patients need special care requiring technical training and skills by a multi-disciplinary team (See Ronald H. Sunderland and Earl E. Shelp, *Handle with Care: A Handbook for Care Teams Serving People with AIDS* [Nashville: Abingdon, 1990]). Often people with AIDS need an HIV Social Worker to arrange housing, medical care, insurance and disability provisions, and professional advocacy.

Offering concrete services such as these is *different from*, not *better than*, offering a ministry of presence. Some are called to *do* something tangible for someone in need; some are called to *be* present to a person's pain. Some may be able to do both.

In the following chapter we will go beyond the basics of care-giving to discuss the skills pastors and professional care-givers need in responding to the needs of people with AIDS.

CHAPTER SEVEN

What to Do When You're Expected to Know What to Do: Issues in Professional and Pastoral Care

"I won't go on. I can't. I know there are people worse off than me. But I know what's ahead. Why postpone the inevitable?"

So, you're a pastor, and someone in your congregation has AIDS. How do you respond? You're a social worker, or a professionally trained care-giver, and you feel helpless in the face of AIDS. What do you do when others expect you to know what to do?

We must recognize that we cannot cure a person with AIDS but we can identify the psychosocial and spiritual issues of AIDS, so that professional and pastoral care can occur either in the hospital setting and in the home. The story of William will serve to raise the issues to which we must be prepared to respond.

Who Am I Without My Books and Things?

William was a young, handsome, intelligent, articulate, good-natured, free-spirited, professional man. His generosity and humor made others feel happy in his company.

Like most young people, William never expected to face death in his thirties. He looked forward to a long, good life. He grew up in a Christian home with a brother and two sisters. He went to church, graduated from college, traveled the world, became a writer, and found employment with a theater company in San Francisco.

134

Life seemed good until his partner was diagnosed with AIDS in the mid 1980s. Reality hit home, and William started to deal with his own mortality and experience of loss. His partner, Richard, eventually died of AIDS. Through testing, William, too, found out he was infected. Yet, he was determined to stay on top of this disease through attention to health, diet, and an exercise program. He had supportive friends, secure employment, adequate insurance, and an apartment filled with foreign books, antique furniture, original art work, and precious things from his travels.

The insidious reality of AIDS struck again in the form of a stroke, and William ended up in the hospital, unable to care for himself. Over the months, he experienced a succession of personal losses that were devastating in every respect.

He had already lost his partner to AIDS. Now he was losing his job and apartment. Most frustrating was his inability to maintain control over his life. Because of his stroke, he was unable to remember things, and often got confused. As dementia began to set in, he actually monitored his loss of mental capacity and became deeply depressed. Eventually, due to a corporate complexity, his company health and disability insurance was canceled, and he had to rely on government programs. Finally, a family decision was made for him to be institutionalized.

All his possessions had to be sold, and his personal assets made available to the system that would support him for the rest of his life. The experience of successive loss devastated William's spirit and rendered him helpless and hopeless, an invalid patient in an institutional hospice unit.

I will never forget visiting William for the first time in his new "home." The building was attractive, and the staff seemed friendly enough. But the institutional atmosphere was dismal. In William's room were three other dying patients. Although the curtain was pulled around William's bed to provide some degree of privacy, there were persistent and distracting coughing, spitting, erratic breathing, and other sounds of sickness.

What to do when you don't know what to do? *Listen!* I sat at bedside and listened for an hour and a half to William, sometimes confused and sometimes coherent, pour out his anguish. With deep groans, sighs and cries, he managed to express some profound existential truths: "Life is so hard, so hard, so very hard. Who am I without my home? Who am I without my books and art? I have some handcrafted books and some personal sketches. All my things are being sold. My life is my books and things. My life is my job and home. My life is my friends, and I've lost everything. There's nothing more to me. My life is defined by the way others see me, by what I have in terms of things, by the work I do and the home I have. It's true, I am my theater company and my books of art. That is who I am . . ."

I was amazed at William's ability to articulate what he felt reduced to—a person without identity or selfhood. I thought of Jesus' teaching about not being anxious about our life, what we will eat, where we will sleep, and what we will wear. For a person's life does not consist of the abundance of his or her possessions (Luke 12:13-34). How beautiful that sounds in the abstract. How difficult for anyone to live out. William looked deep into the abyss, the reality that his life and identity consisted of how he looked, the work he did, where he lived, and what he owned. Confronting the loss of all that defined him, William wept uncontrollably.

What do you do when you're a person of faith who believes that God gives us an essential identity and purpose apart from health, home, job, appearance, and possessions? What do you do as a Christian care-giver when family members expect you to have the answers and to help their child find Christ before he or she dies? You begin by listening to and discussing life and death issues.

DISCUSSING PSYCHOSOCIAL ISSUES

The experience of AIDS and the psychosocial issues that arise are overwhelming: (1) *multiple losses*, (2) *social alienation*, (3) *the stress of living with terminal illness*, (4) *consideration of suicide*, and (5) *progressing through the stages of grief.* Fortunately, there are skills and principles that care-givers can learn to help them be present to and empower the person in need.

Multiple Losses

AIDS patients, in the long and painful course of their disease, experience one loss after another. An AIDS diagnosis may mean loss of physical appearance, loss of sexual contact, loss of health and energy, loss of job and income, loss of home and possessions, loss of friends and family, and loss of personal control over one's own life. The kinds of losses and their severity will differ according to the situation of each individual.

By sitting and listening to a patient's experience of successive loss, the minister or care-giver can remind the person that his or her feelings are all right. If a person who feels deep loss can at least know that another is aware of the pain, the connection itself will bring some relief. This is the power of empathy—when we seek to understand another person's suffering, that person's pain is to some degree diminished.

Empathy means we walk with a person through the valley of the shadow of death, allowing him or her to point out the scenery along the way. The journey is never easy. It's agonizing to watch someone in pain and to feel helpless in the face of it. Physical pain is difficult enough. Mental anguish makes it worse.

The first time I met Bob in the hospital, he was very

self-conscious about the disfigurement on the left side of his face—dark, crusty scabs across his nose and cheek, entangling his mustache. Pointing to his face, he told me: "This is herpes, and I'm resistant to the medication because of AIDS." He told me how embarrassing it's been to go out socially or to explain his condition. "It's not the diagnosis that gets to me," he said. "It's this damn thing on my face and groin." As I tried to hide my internal distress of seeing a once attractive young man suffer the loss of physical appearance, Bob continued to tell me of his loss of job, apartment, roommates, and friends. I felt anguish as I imagined what it might be like if our roles were reversed.

The care-giver's challenge is to stay with the patient's pain as long as possible. We should be present to as much pain as the patient is willing to reveal or we are able to endure. Very few people, including family and friends, can bear to be present to much pain and suffering. Professionals probably can bear to see and hear more pain than most. As the patient reveals his or her life and the pain of multiple losses to the care-giver, a heart-to-heart connection will be made, and God will be present.

Social Alienation

In American society, if you are in the middle to upper class, and are a healthy, law-abiding, white, male heterosexual under the age of fifty-five, you are swimming in the mainstream and will probably be taken care of should you get ill. But if you are poor, a new immigrant, do not speak English, cannot afford insurance, are gay, abuse drugs, or are part of any other subculture, your chances of social alienation are greater.

Gay persons and substance abusers with AIDS often experience social alienation beyond their ability to endure. They are already social outcasts. They may be disenfranchised from family and mainstream contact. When they become ill, the few friends and social provisions they had can quickly disappear.

The experience of social alienation elicits feelings of isolation, abandonment, and despair. These feelings inevitably arise when a person is deprived of social interaction and community. When family members no longer can be supportive, when friends fail to visit, when society stigmatizes, and communities exclude people with AIDS, the result is alienation and despair.

There is a "cure" for feelings of isolation, abandonment, and despair—the gifts of love and acceptance.

After seeing and listening to Bob's mental anguish, I noticed his journal on the table and asked if he were a writer. "Yes," he said, with eyes that suddenly expressed hope. "Would you like to hear a poem I wrote?"

"Certainly," I said.

He read me a beautiful poem about how it is to live with AIDS. The lines themselves and the manner in which he delivered them revealed his depth of emotion, gentle spirit, and compassionate heart. Over the course of several visits, I found myself becoming quite fond of this disfigured young man.

Social isolation is a pain of life that a care-giver can enter into and relieve. If one who cares initiates meaningful interaction, despair will flee. Human interaction brings deep and abiding hope. It is a primary channel that God uses to mediate grace and love.

The Stress of Living with AIDS

Living with AIDS is inherently stressful. The daily routines of eating, dealing with body functions, medical observations, legal concerns, and personal anxiety all contribute to the stress of the disease. How persons perceive, interpret, and understand what is happening to them largely determine the degree of stress and anxiety they will experience. Some persons are more vulnerable than others to the physical and psychological dimensions of stress.

Pastoral and professional care help people with AIDS manage their stress and anxiety. Care begins by simply recognizing and accepting the fact that a person's situation is stressful, and admitting that things probably will continue to be stressful. Rehearsing the facts that have led to anxiety and stress can help prepare a person for the experience of further loss.

Recognizing the *sources* of stress can lead to a discussion of *resources* for coping with stress. Ask your patient what internal and external resources he or she is drawing on for support.

There are resources for hope in the spiritual life, and a patient can be assured that "grace is sufficient" and "hope is available" from God. People with AIDS have proven to themselves and others that they can manage to thrive in spite of serious physical and psychological obstacles. A minister or care-giver can encourage a patient to work on gaining confidence, accessing resources, and building faith to manage the situation.

I went to visit Bob again, hoping for some improvement in his mental state due to the drug treatment he anticipated. The nurse told me Bob was agitated. Nothing seemed to be going right for him. The medication he needed was unavailable, his insurance had run out, and he was being discharged that day. There was nothing we could do.

As I entered Bob's room, he broke into hysteria before I had said a single word. I pulled a chair beside the bed and looked at him with an invitation to tell me about it.

After a long silence on my part, Bob stopped crying and

said, "I can't seem to control it. That's why I don't want to go back to work. What if I broke down on the job? And how do I explain this thing?" (pointing again to the left side of his face).

"Actually, it's looking better than it did last week," I said. "Did you get the medication you needed?"

Picking at the scabs, Bob said, "The lotion the doctor prescribed is not working. The drugs I really need are held up in Washington, D.C. and the authorities are not releasing them for someone like me. It's all very political and very complicated."

"What will you do if you can't get the right medication?"

"I won't go on. I can't. I know there are people worse off than me. But I know what's ahead. I'll lose my job. Without income, I'll lose my apartment. I don't want to go to some AIDS hospice somewhere. Why postpone the inevitable?"

"Do you think you have any inner resources you can draw upon, to keep going? I hate to see you give up so early. What would it take to keep you here?"

"There are a lot of Bobs running around in my head. There are good Bobs and bad Bobs. The bad Bobs are screaming 'Give up!' The good Bobs say 'Live!' Until today, there were enough good Bobs to fight the bad Bobs. But now, there's only one good Bob left. And he's way off on a distant hill with a weak voice that barely floats through the air. It's so faint that the bad Bobs don't even bother to fight him. If they did and the last one good Bob was killed off, I would know it was all over."

I was moved by the image and drama. "So, as long as just one good Bob is alive, you'll stay with us?"

"I guess so."

"Well, I want to encourage the real Bob, the one that's in control, to embrace that one last good Bob in your head. Hold on to him for all you're worth. He represents your inner strength. He is what's keeping you alive. He's your best friend. He's the only hope you have. Will you keep him?"

Bob smiled, "I'll try."

God has not abandoned the one whose strength and hope are gone. There is in every human heart the capacity to receive strength from God to face stress and loss. There is, deep within the human spirit, a wellspring of "hope beyond hope" to be drawn upon. As the Apostle Paul testified in his letter to the Philippians: *"I can do all things I need to do through him [Christ] who gives me strength"* (4:13).

Suicide or Self-deliverance

According to a televised AIDS documentary, "people with AIDS are sixty-six times more likely to commit suicide than the general population." Some of those who end their life are doing so with the help of medical professionals who provide lethal doses of "medication" (KQED, "Wrestling with AIDS," San Francisco, 1989).

Is it morally wrong to commit suicide if you have AIDS? Should doctors, ministers, social workers, and other care-givers try to prevent or help their patients who want to terminate their painful existence? As greater numbers of AIDS patients opt for "self-deliverance," a new slant on an old ethical and religious issue is being raised.

Although I can understand, I personally could not assist a patient who wanted to end his or her life. However, in discussion with other AIDS care-givers and patients, I have learned to appreciate the distinction between "suicide" and "self-deliverance."

Suicide is a quick escape from the pain of life without regard to those one leaves behind. The decision to commit suicide is an isolated, irrational choice based on despair and hopelessness. Family and friends are seldom informed of the decision, and it is carried out alone and in desperation. A person considering suicide believes that "when things get really bad, you can always kill yourself," without regard to the consequences of one's actions on others. Suicide leaves emotional scars on family and friends from which they may never fully recover. Suicide, essentially, is a selfish act based on avoiding relationships.

Self-deliverance, proponents say, is a personal, rational decision carried out in community with others. It is based less on despair and hopelessness, and more on counting the cost of what lies ahead in the disease process. AIDS patients who have watched countless friends and acquaintances die slow and painful deaths have a sense of what their own death will be like. In the face of this inevitability, some AIDS patients explore the options and choose to responsibly shorten the length of their terminal disease.

The ethical considerations of self-deliverance include discussing the impact of such a decision with one's friends and family, considering the feelings and views of others, and being careful not to legally implicate others who might assist.

When an AIDS patient chooses to discuss suicide or self-deliverance with you, there are responsibilities and principles to keep in mind. It is your moral and legal responsibility as a professional member of the health care team to report talk of suicide to your supervisor and/or to your patient's doctor or nurse. Do not keep this information to yourself. If you are a minister, suicide is one issue where you will have to carefully determine whether or not ministerial privilege applies.

It is important to explore the patient's feelings regarding the ending of life. This can be done in a nonjudgmental, supportive way, rather than in a moralistic and imposing manner.

Your role as a care-giver is to *name the reality*: "I hear you saying that you're thinking of ending your life." Your role is to get your patient to talk about the pain behind the desire to end life, and to distinguish the need to relieve the pain from the need to end life. Your role is to relate with the patient in a compassionate way that may alleviate the desire to end life.

If suicide seems to be the clear *intent*, it is your responsibility to determine the *plan* and the *means* the patient has for carrying it out. Ask direct questions: "How and when do you propose to do it?" You might also discuss the risk of failing (most attempts fail) and the possible consequences.

If a patient's mind is made up in favor of self-deliverance, you might challenge him or her to identify the people who need to know, to honestly face them, one by one, and to deal with the impact of the decision with each one before carrying it out.

On my third visit with Bob, we openly discussed suicide, although he did not like to use the term. He informed me that he had discussed the possibility with his doctor, his counselor, and now with me, his chaplain.

"I've thought a lot about this," Bob said intensely. "If I lose my job and become disabled the state will have to take care of me. It will cost a lot of money for hospital care and drug treatments. It's really less selfish for me to save everybody the trouble. If you know what's ahead, then why postpone the inevitable?"

"Have you thought about how you would do it?" I asked.

"Well I certainly wouldn't do it here. I'd do it by myself with no chance of anyone finding me until it was too late. I couldn't stab myself or anything. Too painful. There are other methods, but I'm afraid I'd fail and someone would find me and revive me. I'd probably jump off the Bridge or something."

"Who do you need to contact to inform them of your plans?"

"Well, I guess I should tell my friend, Carl." (We talked a bit about Carl.)

"How about Helen?" (referring to Bob's friend who had become a second mother to him after his natural mother died).

"Oh yes, I must tell Helen not to be surprised."

"Anyone else need to know?"

"No."

I listened again to Bob's long tirades about how tired he was of the "games" in the gay community, about the social elitism, the obsession with beautiful bodies and good looks, the bar and party scene, the dating rituals where people ask for your phone number but never call. "I'm so tired of it all," he moaned. "I don't think I was intended to be gay."

"Bob, I care what happens to you. I hope you will find the reason you are here in this life before your time is up."

"I believe in God, you know," Bob said. "I don't go to church, but I meditate on things. About a life hereafter. I don't know what your beliefs are about suicide [it was the first time he used the word], but I don't think God would blame me."

"God loves you and understands you, Bob. You'll do the right thing. I'm glad you discussed it with me. Personally, I want to encourage you to stay with us. I really enjoy our visits. You have my prayers and blessing."

It was time for me to go. As I rose to leave, Bob got out of bed. "May I have a hug?" I asked.

"Sure, you can have a hug," he said with tears in his eyes. And softly he said, "Good-bye."

I reported our conversation to Bob's doctor, and attempted to follow-up after he was discharged. Bob did not prematurely end his life, but he kept hope alive. Nine months later he was readmitted to the hospital, where he died.

The truth remains: stress, anxiety, alienation, despair, and even suicidal feelings can be honestly faced through the tender loving care of a friend who emotionally connects with a person in pain, and helps to point out resources of help and hope.

Progressing Through the Stages of Grief

I find AIDS patients in general to be deeply spiritual people. Why is this? As a stigmatized and outcast group, people with AIDS easily relate to a God of healing and deliverance. Facing the prospect of an early death, people with AIDS often engage in a new and personal search for spiritual values, meaning, and purpose. They learn to live more deeply, from the center. They often experience the God *who draws near as an ever present help and refuge in time of trouble* (Ps. 46:1).

Many terminally ill people who previously would not have considered themselves particularly religious have a quality of experience and faith that is deeply spiritual.

By the term *spiritual* I mean more than simple orthodoxy of Christian beliefs. I view spirituality similar to the way author John Fortunato defines it in his book, *AIDS: The Spiritual Dilemma:*

> By *spiritual* I allude to the journey of the soul—not to religion itself but the drive in humankind that gives rise to religion in the first place. I have in mind the software on the computer of life, not its hardware; the program as it runs, not the data to be input or the machine that processes it or

146

even the printout. By *spiritual* I am referring to that aura around all of our lives that gives what we do meaning, the human striving toward meaning, the search for a sense of belonging. (pp. 7-8)

What is it in the process of dying that reawakens this dimension of life? Ministers and professional care-givers are aware of the five stages or attitudes toward death and dying, identified by Elisabeth Kübler-Ross, that terminally ill people generally evidence: (1) denial, (2) rage and anger, (3) bargaining, (4) depression, and (5) acceptance. *(On Death and Dying* [New York: Macmillan, 1969]). In each stage of terminal illness, there are appropriate times and ways to raise spiritual issues and witness the reality of God at work in a life.

Denial:

"Not me!"

To deny that one is sick and dying may be at first a healthy sign. As a defense mechanism, denial cushions the impact that death may be imminent. For example, if a person who is HIV positive believes that he or she will not get sick and die, it is inappropriate to confront the patient's denial with the fact that most people with AIDS die within a few years. As Jack Pantaleo, founder of the San Francisco AIDS Interfaith Network, notes: "I used to believe that telling people that they might live was instilling false hope. Now I believe that if I expect people to die, it gives them false despair."

The pastor's and professional care-giver's task during the denial stage is to gently encourage and support the patient in the process of dealing with the new reality. God is present in *denial* as the One who gives faith and hope against all odds.

147

Rage and Anger:
"Why me?"

Unless there is physical healing or remission, denial of the disease process gradually gives way to anger and rage. "Why is this happening to me?" the patient demands to know. The question is put to God, to the church, to the medical team, and to anyone who will listen.

The care-giver's task is to simply sit and listen. A patient may need to express the resentment about why others remain alive and healthy while he or she must die. Angry, enraged, and dying patients, in the words of Dylan Thomas, "do not go gentle into that good night but rage, rage, against the dying of the light" ("Do Not Go Gentle into That Good Night").

God is always a special target for rage and anger since God is thought to be the One who indiscriminately punishes and arbitrarily imposes the death sentence. Ministers and priests are also singled out for verbal abuse because they represent the church, which has so often failed to love, accept, and forgive the "sinner."

The spiritual task, I repeat, is not to debate the nature of God or to defend the church, but *to sit and take it on the chin!* In listening to rage and anger poured out upon us, we represent the God of all compassion who patiently listens to the children of creation pour out their anguished hearts in prayer.

Bargaining:
"I'll make you a deal"

The next stage or attitude in coping with terminal illness is trying to bargain with God. "If you heal me, God, I will join a monastery." "If you grant me five more years, I will serve you among the poor." "If you give me one more chance, I will never have sex again." People who, prior to their illness, never prayed to God suddenly make all sorts of promises and strike all kinds of bargains.

The pastoral task at this stage is *not* to exploit the spiritual vulnerability of the patient by soliciting a confession and commitment, but rather to represent the God who does not bargain but simply wants us all to come home.

The story of the prodigal son illustrates this point: "I'll bargain with my father," the son said to himself. "Perhaps he'll let me be one of his hired hands." But the father was not interested in striking bargains. Instead, he called for a celebration, "for my son was lost and now is found."

Depression:

"Woe is me"

Bargaining gradually gives way to depression, signaling the recognition that the end is near. Sometimes called "preparatory grief," depression brings the awareness of impending separation and loss. AIDS patients often speak of "losing ground" and "giving into the process." There is no more denial of approaching death. There is sadness and despondency, sometimes relief, a closing of relationships, a completing of personal business.

The pastoral task is to listen to how the patient is dealing with the hard questions. As chaplains, we can then pose these same questions in an open-ended manner to help them verbalize what is going on inside. We can ask: Where are you regarding making peace with the past? Does anything need to be done for you to be at peace with family and friends? Are you at peace with yourself and with your God? Is there anyone you need to forgive? Have you forgiven yourself? Do you know God's love and forgiveness? Are you ready to cross over to the other side?

Often, there is still unfinished business to complete,

relationships to reconcile, and personal arrangements to make. Beyond the practical concerns of reviewing and detaching from one's estate, preparing or updating one's will, and planning one's funeral and burial—which themselves raise difficult feelings and emotion-laden issues—a dying person is also concerned about closure with family and friends.

Ministers and care-givers can be spiritually helpful in facilitating the farewells. Pastoral care not only empowers a person to make peace with the past, but helps a person deal with the present and prepare for the future. When the hard work of this stage is accomplished, the gift of *acceptance* is given.

Acceptance:

"It's okay that my time has come"

Acceptance is not necessarily a happy stage. But neither is it an unhappy one. It is not a helpless resignation to the inevitable. It is more like a personal victory, a spiritual triumph over the fear of death. As death draws near, the patient might be able to identify with the Apostle Paul, who said, "The time has come for my departure. I have fought the good fight, I have finished the race, I have kept the faith. Now there is in store for me the crown of righteousness" (II Tim. 4:6-8).

Not all AIDS patients embrace the end stage with peace and acceptance. Many die ugly and chaotic deaths. Some continue to "rage against the dying of the light" until their last, dying breath. Some defy all categories and stages of death and dying.

But with those who die at peace with God, there seems to be a pattern. After their last "good-bye," they start to slip away. Their eyes turn inward to gaze beyond the vale of tears to the light beyond. Their spirits sail to the other shore, and then return, bringing assurance that God is waiting for them on the other side. And when the moment of transition occurs at death's cold door, a song of the soul set free can be heard in the heart: "It is well with my soul. / It is well, it is well with my soul."

The Terrible yet Tender Death of Eugene

"Eugene is dying," the nurse told me. "He wants to see a priest."

As the chaplain on duty, I went into Eugene's room and introduced myself. He was literally bleeding to death, coughing up blood, urinating blood, and bleeding from lesions. "Say a prayer for me, Father," he managed to say.

I asked him if he were ready to cross over. He said, "Yes, I've made my peace, and I've seen heaven."

"What's it like?" I asked.

"Well, it's hard to say; can't really explain it."

"I'm glad you're ready. God is waiting for you."

Eugene smiled. He started to cough up more blood. I recoiled. He apologized. I placed my hand on his brow and made the sign of the cross. I prayed a prayer of commendation to God, that Eugene's spirit would be received with joy on the other side. His partner sat there silently in tears.

Though anxious to leave this world behind, Eugene hung on for several days. He finally stopped bleeding, went unconscious, and quietly died. The nurses commented about the peace he had in passing. I knew in my heart that he had drunk from the stream of living water and would be with Christ on the other side.

AIDS patients who have made peace with God and accepted their impending death have much to teach us about healing, overcoming fear, and putting our hope in God.

CHAPTER EIGHT

A Light Burning in the Darkness:
The Ministry of Healing and Hope

"When Mother Teresa was in town, she came to visit me in the hospital. I thought it was during my third bout with pneumonia. I thought I was going to die. She touched my forehead and said I would recover. I did, without any of those drugs they use to keep people alive."

Do miracles happen with AIDS? Do people get cured of terminal diseases? What does the Church of Jesus Christ—which believes in God's power to heal and restore human lives—have to offer people living with AIDS?

I believe God can heal people physically as well as spiritually. However, to the best of my knowledge, no actual, verifiable physical healing of AIDS has occurred. There have been people in remission, HIV-positive people free of symptoms, but I do not know of any miracle cures.

On the other hand, inner emotional and spiritual healing is common in AIDS ministry. On numerous occasions I have witnessed the power of God, in response to prayers of faith, raise a person up in body, soul, and spirit, and restore that person to life and wholeness. This is the kind of healing that this chapter celebrates.

"Sybil Doesn't Live Here Anymore"

LeRoy James Bennett III, a young, handsome, outgoing gay man from a middle-class black family, was diagnosed with AIDS in 1986. He has survived three bouts with pneumocystis pneumonia (PCP), four hospitalizations, and is allergic to most of the recommended drug treatments, including AZT, which slow the disease's progress. I asked him how he managed to stay alive for so long. "My faith in God," he replied with the sparkle of hope in his eyes.

LeRoy was raised a Christian in the Pentecostal tradition. Early in life he was called to preach. Resisting the call, he became a musician in San Francisco. Years of roaming with the wrong crowd, drug abuse, and anonymous sex took their toll, and LeRoy came down with AIDS.

"I did everything there is to do," he admitted. "Then the Lord got a hold on me and brought me back to faith. Now I'm back in church, singing with the youth choir. I'm warning them about AIDS. Last month I gave my testimony before the whole congregation. I'm not the preacher I was meant to be, but the Lord has given me a ministry."

I was deeply moved by LeRoy's testimony. His story was one of healing and deliverance, not from being homosexual, but from living the gay life in the fast lane apart from God. He didn't expect God to completely heal him of AIDS, but he did have the faith to believe that God would keep him alive and well until his work was done.

I asked LeRoy what work he had to finish before it was time to go. He showed me the book he was writing entitled *Sybil Doesn't Live Here Anymore.* "It's my life story and testimony of faith and healing," he said proudly. No longer was he leading a chaotic, schizophrenic life.

He shared with me one dramatic healing episode: "When Mother Teresa was in town, she came to visit me in the hospital. It was during my third bout with pneumonia. I thought I was going to die. She touched my forehead and said I would recover. I did, without any of those drugs they use to keep people alive."

LeRoy said he no longer feared death, "because I know my grandmother is waiting for me to take me to heaven."

Every time I saw LeRoy, his faith was strong. Even when his body was weak, he was able to claim God's healing hand on his life until it was his time to go. I learned much from LeRoy about God's power to sustain the body and heal the spirit.

153

LeRoy's testimony reveals at least three principles of divine healing: (1) healing happens even when there is no permanent cure; (2) prayer is good for your health; and (3) living with AIDS has spiritually healing benefits.

HEALING WHERE THERE IS NO CURE

A poignant prophecy is found in Talmudic literature. A young rabbi is asking an older rabbi, "Where will we find Messiah?" The older rabbi responds: "You will find Messiah, when he comes, outside the gates of the city changing the bandages of the lepers."

Matthew's Gospel records,

> When John [the Baptist] heard in prison what Jesus was doing, he sent his disciples to ask him, "Are you the one who was to come, or should we expect someone else?" Jesus replied, "Go back and report to John what you hear and see: The blind receive sight, the lame walk, those who have leprosy are cured, the deaf hear, the dead are raised, and the good news is preached to the poor." (Matt. 11:2-5)

Jesus of Nazareth demonstrated that he was the Messiah by embracing the poor, accepting the outcasts, forgiving the sinners, and healing the sick with power and authority.

The Gospels record that Jesus healed many lepers in response to simple faith (Matt. 8:1-3). When Jesus was in Bethany, he and his disciples ate in the home of Simon the leper. Jesus was not afraid to "recline at table," the most intimate form of socializing in his time, with someone who had a contagious disease (Mark 14:3).

On another occasion, ten people with leprosy came to Jesus with a request: "Have mercy on us" (Luke 17:12-19). Jesus did not predicate his willingness to heal them on their repentance of their sins or even their commitment to become disciples. He simply responded to their appeal for mercy. All ten lepers were healed—unconditionally! Only one of them returned and thanked Jesus for healing him. The one grateful leper, who threw himself at Jesus' feet and worshiped him, was a Samaritan! Jesus' willingness to heal had no conditions; he healed the lepers simply because they believed. Even Samaritan lepers were not beyond his healing touch.

Jesus commissioned his disciples to go among the outcasts of Israel and preach to them that the kingdom of God was near. He told them not only to preach the good news but to demonstrate its power: "Heal the sick, raise the dead, cleanse those who have leprosy, drive out demons. Freely you have received, freely give" (Matt. 10:8). Again, Jesus did not say that the outcasts of Israel had to repent and believe before they were embraced and healed. Rather, Jesus told his disciples to go in his name, and that any who received them with hospitality and gratitude were in fact receiving the Messiah (Matt. 10:40).

The kind of "evangelism" Jesus practiced and taught his followers was that of embracing and healing social outcasts. How does the church's imperative to embrace and heal the lost apply to people with AIDS?

In San Francisco, during the early years of the AIDS epidemic, a small group of courageous Christians, desiring to see the church respond with compassion, met for prayer every Wednesday morning for a year on the steps of Grace Cathedral. They prayed for the churches to open their doors and offer healing services for people with AIDS.

Roman Catholic Archbishop John Quinn responded by inviting AIDS patients and ministers of all faiths to participate in a marathon weekend of prayer and healing. The sick would be anointed with oil and prayed for by a "laying-on of hands." Six hundred people attended the special ceremony called "Forty Hours Devotion"—revived from the medieval liturgy first invoked in the fourteenth century in Italy when thousands were dying of the Black Death. The liturgy offered a sign of hope in a city where forty persons with AIDS were dying every month. A new ministry, known as the AIDS Interfaith Network, evolved out of the "Forty Hours Devotion" and the prophetic weekly prayer meetings that preceded it. Under the leadership of Jack Pantaleo, the Network initiated and cosponsored four healing services each month in San Francisco—in the Episcopal, Unitarian Universalist, Metropolitan Community Church, and Pentecostal traditions.

Several years have passed since those early healing services. Today, only one monthly AIDS healing service remains from the original four. The Episcopal churches now incorporate the need for AIDS healing in their regular services. The Unitarian Universalist service was never well attended and eventually ceased to be held. The Pentecostal healing service initially was quite popular and well attended. The fervency of prayers, the emotionally charged worship experience, and the strong belief in physical healing resulted in several cases of reported healing and deliverance. Unfortunately, the pastor who responded to the need for a healing service and was willing to suspend moral judgments about homosexuality was criticized by more conservative ministers who questioned whether healing should be offered to those who did not "repent of homosexual sin." The pastor relocated to another church, and the healing service eventually was discontinued.

Only the AIDS healing service at Metropolitan Community Church, San Francisco (MCC-SF) continued to thrive on a monthly basis. Though controversial, it remains a compelling model of *compassionate, inclusive,* and *unconditional* healing ministry in the spirit of Jesus.

WE ARE A CHURCH WITH AIDS

MCC-SF is an inclusive church of 300 members, with over 500 in weekly attendance. Most of the parishioners are homosexual. About two thirds of the men in the congregation are HIV positive or have AIDS. The pastor's vision for the church is that "it should be a house of prayer for all people."

MCC-SF is part of a larger denomination founded in 1969 by the Reverend Troy Perry, a former Pentecostal minister. Today, the Universal Fellowship of Metropolitan Community Churches consists of 249 congregations in 13 countries representing over 30,000 members, mostly gay and lesbian.

Rejected by established churches and traditions because of their homosexuality, many gay Christians find an outlet for their faith in Metropolitan Community Churches. At MCC-SF, a decade of living with AIDS has sparked a spiritual renewal resulting in unprecedented growth and expansion of services.

"We have come to understand ourselves as a church with AIDS," says Jim Mitulski, the church's senior pastor.

> This doesn't mean that our church will soon be dead and gone. No, in fact it means we live more deeply. The whole gay male community is undergoing a parallel transformation. A life-style characterized by carefree promiscuity has given way to dating and friendship. Many people are seeking intimacy and spirituality, which has had the effect of a revival.[1]

It is difficult to capture the experience of worshiping in a "gay church." My wife and I were first invited to attend a service in November 1988. Rebecca had met the pastor in a

---

[1] "We Are the Church Alive, the Church with AIDS," by Kittridge Cherry and James Mitulski, *Christian Century* (January 27, 1988).

class they were both taking at a local seminary. As they became friends, he invited our AIDS Mission Group to a Sunday night "worship and praise" AIDS healing service. Twenty-five Nazarenes, including our district superintendent and his wife and a denominational representative from Kansas City, were welcomed with grateful and sustained applause by a warm and enthusiastic congregation of 200 members on Thanksgiving Sunday evening.

The service opened with prayer, familiar hymns and choruses. Despite our initial discomfort (the idea of gay persons worshiping God was a new concept to many in our group), we all felt at home with the spirited singing and familiar selections by the gospel choir, led by a former Baptist who played the piano with exceptional style. The worship team also included musicians on pipe organ, drums, guitar, and bass.

There were heartfelt testimonies punctuated with "Praise God!" and "Hallelujah!" Some gave testimony of deliverance from drugs and alcohol. Others simply said "thank you God" for life and health or some blessing during the week. It reminded me of an old-fashioned Nazarene camp meeting—hands waving in the air, tears welling up in the eyes of the redeemed, exuberant praise and worship of a God who saves and sanctifies.

The Scriptures were read, and then the altar area was opened for a time of healing prayer. We as honored guests were asked to join those at the altar to pray through the laying-on of hands for those who had AIDS.

Dozens responded, including a frail young man with AIDS in the second row who literally leaped out of his seat and ran into our healing circle. Sobbing, he poured out his soul. Asking for a special touch of God, we embraced his thin, crippled frame and prayed for healing. About fifteen to twenty people affected by AIDS requested and received prayer with the laying-on of hands, hoping for a healing touch from God.

Did anyone get *physically* healed? I am aware of none. But *inner* healing happened, and people with AIDS found new faith and strength to keep going and to stay on top of their disease.

Other broken and hurting persons from many walks of life came forward, requesting healing from sexual abuse or prayer for self-acceptance. One woman I prayed with asked for release from early childhood scars, including the trauma of incest. Another woman, a first-time visitor, asked to be healed of her fear of gay persons. A young man confessed that he had been emotionally and physically abused and requested healing "for my inner child."

During the prayer time, the choir sang "In This Very Room."

The service was also a time of repentance and healing for the Nazarenes in attendance. We represented all those who had inflicted (perhaps unknowingly) the emotional pain of ridicule and rejection. I thought of gay people I had known whom I had devalued or subtly rejected. I thought of the Lord wanting all his children to live in peace, loving each other as neighbors. I was conscious that we were standing on holy ground, and that God was much bigger than what I had previously thought. I noticed that I was not the only one so moved, for there were very few dry eyes in the congregation.

Holy Communion followed as the culmination of the worship and healing experience. As parishioners lined up to receive the cup and bread, tears were shed, hugs were exchanged, hands were raised in response to what was happening in church. God Almighty was undeniably present with healing power from on high.

The two-and-a-half-hour service ended with everyone

holding hands around the sanctuary, praying and singing together the familiar hymn "It Is Well with My Soul." I was emotionally drained, spiritually charged, and profoundly touched by what took place. There was much on which to reflect and apply to AIDS ministry.

Our District Superintendent, Clarence Kinzler, later summarized what we all felt: "I don't know what to think about it all, but I know Jesus was there. And because Jesus was there, that's where we should be."

He also said that he found himself repenting of how he and one of his previous congregations had treated a gay member. "We just didn't know what to do with him."

Several former Nazarenes warmly introduced themselves to us after the service. One young woman with joy in her eyes said to Pastor Kinzler after the service, "Do you know how long it's been since I've talked to a Nazarene minister, much less a district superintendent? Thank you for coming to my church!" We were all amazed by the number of men and women who joined MCC and who came from conservative evangelical backgrounds. Many had rejection stories to tell. We stood, as a congregation, convicted by our own prejudice.

After our shared experience at Metropolitan Community Church, I sensed from my district superintendent permission to care for persons with AIDS without judgment, to build a bridge of love, acceptance, and forgiveness to gay people who have felt abandoned by the church. "Some of our own Nazarene boys are out there, and we've got to let them know we love them," Pastor Kinzler said. He also challenged us to walk the line between acceptance of persons and endorsement of life-style, and added: "While we're not *pro-gay*, we are *pro-people*."

Members of the Metropolitan Community Church, which accepts homosexuality as a special gift of God to be integrated into one's life of faith, found it hard to believe that members of the Church of the Nazarene, which officially condemns homosexuality as sin, would even step foot inside their sanctuary, much less join them for worship. These two seemingly irreconcilable traditions managed to put theological, moral, and rejection issues aside for a couple of hours and find common ground in praying for persons with AIDS. No longer was AIDS an issue of "us" and "them." Together, we knew ourselves to be the body of Christ; we knew ourselves as the church with AIDS.

Several of us continued attending the monthly AIDS healing services at MCC-SF. In so doing, we not only brought spiritual healing by our presence and participation, but we ourselves were becoming healed of our prejudices toward gay persons and our opinions about AIDS.

One member of our AIDS Mission Group, Muriel Beukelman, at sixty-three years of age adopted MCC-SF as her mission field for a year. On weekdays, she visited those with AIDS and offered a ministry of healing and hope. On Sunday nights, she sang in the church choir and was adopted by many in the congregation as a surrogate mother. Gay persons estranged from family often are in need of love and acceptance. Muriel offered motherly love and became a human instrument of God's power to heal and restore.

How God Prepared Me for AIDS Ministry
by Muriel Beukelman

When I first came to San Francisco, and joined the staff of Golden Gate Ministries, my work was with the homeless. Two years later, an AIDS Mission Group was formed, and I joined. As some of us began to visit people with AIDS, I slowly realized God wanted me to love these people and to try to build a bridge connecting them with God.

Many of those God called me to love and accept were homosexuals. I was uncomfortable at first, but in getting to know them as individuals, and realizing that they too were God's beloved children, I came to enjoy their company.

I was invited to attend the AIDS healing service at MCC on Thanksgiving evening. What I found was a very warm and loving community. Prayers were prayed for healing, and songs were sung affirming faith in God. There were many tears shed and praises to God. My heart was broken by the terrible plight of those with AIDS and by their strong faith in God's love and healing power. I didn't understand how a person could be a homosexual and a Christian at the same time, but I couldn't refute God's Spirit in that service and in those people.

I decided to attend the Sunday evening services as often as possible. God led me to sing with their choir and to join their AIDS ministry team. I've attended MCC for nearly a year now, and I have made some dear and wonderful friends. I am loved and affirmed by the members of MCC to an almost embarrassing degree.

I marvel at how God prepared me for this kind of ministry. I had an unhappy childhood, deprived of my mother's love because of her emotional illness. My marriage ended in divorce after my husband of twenty years left me. I had five children who were college age in the 1960s, which taught me a measure of tolerance. I believe that the rejection I felt as a child, a wife, and a mother sensitized me to the pain and rejection suffered by my homosexual and lesbian friends. This has given me a degree of understanding of who they are and why.

Homosexuals and people with AIDS have stories filled with pain. I believe God is calling us to love and support them. God is not calling us to judge them, for only God can do that.

When Muriel's year of ministry was completed, she decided to move on to another mission field—that of intercessory prayer in a monastic community. Her farewell service at MCC-SF was a profoundly moving celebration of her commitment to the congregation and her ministry of healing and hope. After the choir sang a tribute—"We Are Standing on Holy Ground"—Muriel was asked to say a few words:

> God has given me a great love for all of you. When I first started coming here a year ago, I was afraid that since I am straight and about the same age as your mothers, you might shut your hearts to me and not trust me. Instead, you have loved and accepted me so completely that I feel like a full member of the congregation. I appreciate that. Whatever good you see in me is Jesus. And the beauty and goodness I see in you, I know it's Jesus. So let us lift up Jesus so that all will be drawn to him for salvation and healing.

"BUT LORD, THEY'RE GAY!"

Some readers, undoubtedly, will question the legitimacy of a church like MCC-SF being held up as a model of compassionate, inclusive, and unconditional healing ministry in the AIDS crisis. Homosexuality is an issue that frequently divides the church and society into liberal and conservative camps. Since homosexuality has been closely related to the spread of HIV infection in the United States, we should discuss the issue openly, with honesty and courage.

Is homosexuality a sin or a constitutional orientation? Can homosexuals change and become heterosexuals? Are "healing" and "deliverance" possible for the person who has known only (or primarily) same-sex attractions and relationships?

After years of pastoral involvement with gay persons, I have come to accept the scientific findings that suggest that homosexual tendencies are a given, constitutional reality for 5 to 10 percent of the population, and that the church is not exempt from this occurrence. People are born and raised in society at large and in the church in particular who are naturally inclined toward same-sex relationships. The reasons—biological, chemical, psychological, or sociological—for this inclination vary depending on the studies one believes.

Instead of trying to understand a homosexual person's struggle for sexual identity, the church generally has responded with rejection. What happens when children of God who are homosexual are forced to live with rejection? Some reject the church and seek the opposite extreme by living promiscuous, empty lives. Others attempt to be straight, hoping their secret desires are never discovered. Many, after years of alienation and rejection, join affirming and reconciling congregations where their homosexuality will be accepted. Some find their way back to traditional churches, hoping to be accepted for who they really are.

When homosexual persons become Christians, or return to the church after years of living without a faith community, they embrace a personal relationship with Jesus Christ. Some are able to live celibate lives. Some are able to marry an understanding spouse, and attempt to live a heterosexual life and raise a family. Some, for psychological and emotional health, opt for a loving and committed same-sex partner, seeking to integrate their sexuality and their spirituality. Very few are "cured" through ex-homosexual ministries.

Inner healing does happen, for the homosexual and for the heterosexual with emotional wounds. But healing is an individual matter. It is not our place to prescribe but God's to determine how and when healing occurs. Nor is it our job to judge. But it is the Holy Spirit's work to convict and cleanse all from sin.

Despite the judgmental rhetoric of self-righteous critics, compassionate Christians know that God loves, accepts, forgives, and saves all who call upon Jesus' name. There is a place in the kingdom and in the church for all God's children.

While we do not have to agree theologically with other believers, or condone life-styles that we find morally objectionable, we should not, through rejection and ridicule, exclude from God's kingdom or the Church anyone who knows God and bears fruit in his or her attitudes and life. Our doctrine of the Church Universal—a historic and biblical doctrine of inclusivity and mutuality in Christ—forbids us to require more (or less) of people than what Christ required to follow him. By embracing those who feel like outcasts, and including them in the community of faith, *healing happens even when the cure is not found.*

PRAYER IS GOOD FOR YOUR HEALTH

The second healing principle to celebrate is that prayer is good for your health and well-being. Medical science has finally verified what the church has always known. According to a nine-month study conducted at San Francisco General Hospital and summarized in the *Journal of the American Medical Association,* heart patients have fewer medical problems when other people pray for their recovery (*San Francisco Chronicle,* January 24, 1989).

Irene Smith, a massage therapist and hospice volunteer, believes in "healing through touch" and founded an organization by that name. She and her volunteers hold out healing hands to the sick and dying, gently massaging them with compassion and touching them with love. Her healing method works, for it reaches the spirit as well as the body. It reduces pain as well as gives comfort. It dispels confusion as well as brings joy. It counters feelings of isolation as well as relieves frazzled nerves. Above all, human touch takes people to a new depth of awareness of inner resources.

Prayer and *human touch* are the ingredients of any healing ministry. The Epistle of James describes the ancient church's ritual for healing prayer: "Is any one of you sick? He should call for the elders of the church to pray over him and anoint him with oil in the name of the Lord. And the prayer offered in faith will make the sick man well, and the Lord will raise him up. If he has sinned, he will be forgiven" (James 5:14-15).

There are many ways to enact this healing provision. In the Roman Catholic tradition, the Anointing of the Sick is one of the seven sacraments of the church. It can be offered by a priest in church, in the home, or in the hospital. Catholic hospital chaplains carry a small vial of holy oil for the purpose of touching, anointing, and praying for patients who desire to be healed.

In the Protestant tradition, ministers as well as laity are empowered to anoint with oil, lay on hands, and pray for people's healing. Some charismatic churches believe that the prayer of faith almost guarantees that the one who claims healing will be healed. Other churches have learned to boldly pray for healing while adding to their intention "not my will, but Thine be done."

The common thread in each tradition is the belief that people can be healed in response to faith, and that God is the One who heals in partnership with those willing to reach out, touch, and pray.

There are several types of healing services that can be offered by any church or ministry team that believes in the Healing Spirit. A few varieties include *healing circles*, where a small group surrounds, touches, prays for, and empowers a person; *eucharistic healing*, where the sacrament of anointing is offered as part of a Communion service; *ecumenical healing*, where the Healing Spirit is invoked through different religious traditions and practices; *guided meditations*, where reflective music, artwork, and visualization techniques are used to access inner spiritual resources; and *healing through praise and worship*, where the power of corporate praise and devotion is unleashed to raise people's spirits, healing body and soul.

The most meaningful AIDS healing service I attended was sponsored by the San Francisco AIDS Interreligious Coalition in anticipation of the International AIDS Conference in San Francisco. Representatives from five religious traditions led the service. A Roman Catholic priest from the Cathedral read from the lectionary and commented on its significance in time of AIDS. A pastor from the Swedenborgian church offered a sacred reading and lit a candle as a petition for healing power to be present that night. A Zen Buddhist chanted in solidarity with all suffering beings. I, an evangelical, affirmed the Christian belief in divine healing and offered a homily. Finally, a Jewish Rabbi led prayers.

People with AIDS in the congregation were invited to come forward, not to be healed but to lead the healing. As four clusters of persons with AIDS took their positions at four points of the compass, signifying a cross, the rest of the congregation was invited to come forward to be healed. I found my way to a cluster and requested a special healing touch of God for my emotional stress and burnout. My heart was warmed as I, the physically healthy one, received the laying-on of hands by a frail, terminally ill healer. As I reflected on this sacramental moment, I was reminded that healing flows both ways; that the one who offers healing is both healer and the healed; and that God as the Healing Spirit desires to heal all, whether or not we have AIDS.

LIVING WITH AIDS HAS HIDDEN GIFTS

The third healing principle has to do with the quality of life available to the person living with AIDS.

My good friend Stanley, unable to get out of bed after surviving a bout with pneumonia, phoned me with constructive criticism concerning the name of our new ministry. From his perspective, the name "Living with AIDS" was an oxymoron: "You call this living? I can't return to work. I can't fend for myself. Some days I don't want to get up. Some days I want to stay down. Call it 'Coping with AIDS' if you want, but not 'Living with AIDS.' " Although I could have easily written off Stanley's comments as expressions of a bad day, I listened and learned and took his comments to heart.

Care-givers must be careful not to impose their optimism on people who are suffering. It does no good to say to someone sick and dying, "You can learn to live with this"; or "All things work together for good"; or "Every cloud has a silver lining." It is a patient's right to interpret his or her physical experience with illness and to draw conclusions about any good that can possibly result.

Having made this essential qualification, I wish to affirm the biblical truth that "in all things, God works for the good" (Rom. 8:28), but not all things are good. Even when terrible and tragic things happen, like an AIDS diagnosis, there are gifts and graces that can be found in them. It is in this context, then, that one may find the dark clouds passing and the sun appearing to inspire persons *living with AIDS.*

Many people who are suffering and living with AIDS have testified to others that were it not for this awful disease, they would not have found God. Others have shared miraculous stories of how they found love, peace, and reconciliation with family through AIDS.

Father John, who directs Kairos House, a support and resource center for AIDS care-givers in San Francisco, offered the following Christmas meditation for those who were able to see beyond the pain and embrace the hidden gifts of AIDS.

The Gifts of AIDS

For many of us affected by the AIDS epidemic, this year's holiday gatherings may be times when we are reminded of "who's missing," and we may re-experience our grief and loss. However, the holidays are traditionally associated with giving, and if we can look beyond the pain, we may find some gifts hidden in the shadows.

Intimacy. Think of someone who has been drawn into your life, or you into theirs, as a result of AIDS. Think of the sharings that have occurred . . . including the tears, the fear, the pain . . . how the facade was stripped away and the humanness of each of you made vulnerable and available to the other. Has the gift of intimacy opened your heart to greater acceptance of yourself and others?

Surrender. Think of some instance where you had to let go of your need for control. Perhaps it was letting go of denial and surrendering to the painful truth of the diagnosis of someone you love. Perhaps you also had to surrender the need to change or fix or cure that person. Perhaps you had to surrender to a changing relationship or let go of it altogether. Or it may have been letting go of an activity or habit. Perhaps you had to surrender to caring for another, or yourself. How has the gift of surrender given you the opportunity to relax a little more deeply into the mystery of life?

Community. Think of a bridge that has been built in your life as a result of AIDS. Perhaps it connected you with someone across the gap of a difference in sexual orientation. Perhaps it was establishing a connection with a support group, a service organization, or healing circle. Perhaps it was reaching out to a new ethnic group, learning about a different spiritual tradition, or connecting with a family member. The gift of community has grown out of our common cause and our compassionate response. How has the gift of community expanded your sense of connectedness?

Service. Think of something you do for another or allow another to do for you as a result of AIDS. The gift of service melts giving and receiving into one act of love. Receiving is giving and giving is receiving. How has the gift of service opened you to a greater appreciation of our interdependence?

Wisdom. Think of something you have learned because of AIDS. Perhaps it is something about the miraculous complexity of our bodies, or maybe it is something about courage and endurance, about love and relationships, about ethics and values. How has the gift of wisdom expanded your awareness?

Presence. Think of some moment where you were with yourself or with another as a result of AIDS where you were totally present. Where the intensity of the moment moved you so deeply that past and future suddenly faded away and all of you responded, resonated with the power of that moment. How has the gift of presence enabled you to live more completely in the now?

Meaning. Think of some aspect of life that has new meaning for you as a result of AIDS: relationships . . . career . . . the arts . . . political process . . .

. . . spirituality. How has the gift of meaning changed your values, your perspective of life, including death?

Love. Think of some expression of love as a result of AIDS that moved you. Some unexpected evidence of love that surpassed all of your expectations. Perhaps it was something that whelmed up within you, or it may have been something that flowed to you in a sharing or gesture. Perhaps it is the compassion and creativity so evident in our response to the epidemic. How has the gift of love touched you at the core of your being?

Intimacy, surrender, service, wisdom, presence, meaning, love. . . . These are the opportunities of our crisis, the silver lining of a dark cloud, the gifts of AIDS to be remembered this holiday season along with those missing friends and loved ones.[2]

Healing happens even when there is no cure. Prayer works wonders in the age of AIDS, and God works for good *in all things,* even in the hidden gifts that come from living with AIDS.

---

[2] *Together We Care,* 2, no. 11 (December 1989).

CHAPTER NINE

The Light at the End of the Tunnel: Compassionate Ministry as Death Draws Near

"I'm going to die today. I love you, I love you all."

Eight-year-old Benny died of AIDS in 1987. CBS made a movie about the trauma called "Moving Toward the Light."

As the child lies dying in his mother's arms, he asks: "What will it be like?"

She whispers softly in his ear: "You will see a light, Benny, far away—a beautiful, shining light at the end of a long tunnel. And your spirit will lift up out of your body and start to travel toward the light. And as you go, a veil will be lifted from your eyes, and suddenly, you'll see everything. . . . But most of all, you will feel a tremendous sense of love."

"Will it take long?"

"No, Benny, not long at all. Like the twinkling of an eye . . ."

This is a chapter on death and dying. It explores how some AIDS patients *face the fear of death,* and in the process, find faith and hope in the Light beyond the grave. It describes how many people with AIDS *prepare to cross over* by taking care of unfinished business and by finally letting go in response to permission from those they leave behind. This chapter also recommends a program for *pastoral care at the time of death* as well as an invitation to *face your own mortality* and *visualize your own death.*

FACING THE FEAR OF DEATH

Every day, thousands of people die. Some die of natural causes and old age. Some die young due to accidents, violent crimes, drugs, suicide, or diseases such as AIDS.

Though death is a part of life, society has gone to great lengths to help us avoid the subject. We soften the language of death: "Grandpa expired"; "Peter passed away." We seal caskets or make sure the corpse we view looks lifelike. We try to shelter our children and ourselves from the reality of death. Death and dying are simply unpleasant subjects for discussion and too threatening to embrace in ministry.

It is natural to be afraid of death and dying. Psychologists tell us it is really not death we fear, but the pain of death and what death symbolizes. Death and dying represent extinction, being alone, separation from those we love, physical pain as well as the pain of not realizing one's purpose and potential, accountability and judgment in the hands of God, and transition into the great unknown.

When terminal issues are addressed by care-givers, especially by those who have faced their own mortality and have hope beyond the grave, there is the possibility that those who face death can do so without isolation and despair. Dying can be experienced as a transition to that place of no pain. Death can be seen as the gateway to rebirth, the promise of Light at the end of the tunnel.

"That's All I Need to Know"

Arnold truly is a remarkable man—witty, intelligent, good-natured, humorous, and outgoing. Born in Virginia, he has a southern drawl and talks nonstop about his daddy's business, his personal life history, his coming of age in the 70s, his Nazarene church background, and many other matters. Finally, I ask if I may pull up a chair and sit down.

"Of course," he answers, and suddenly changes the tenor of the conversation. "I'm sorry for rambling on for so long. Maybe I'm avoiding the business I've got to deal with."

"What business is that?" I inquire.

"I need to tell my family about my diagnosis. My father is seventy years old, and my brother is younger than I am. I don't know how to tell them."

"How do you think they will respond?" I ask.

"My father will just die. My brother won't want to see me."

"I bet you they'll both want to see you. Why don't you find out?"

"I guess I will." Suddenly, Arnold decides to call his father collect in Virginia. He wants me to stay in the room with him while he makes the call.

"Hello, Daddy. This is Arnold . . . I'm in the hospital . . . Daddy, I have AIDS. . . . I HAVE AIDS!"

Arnold is crying uncontrollably. His father is apparently shocked and saying that there is nothing he could do about it. Regaining self-control, Arnold continues talking: "I don't want you to do anything about it, Daddy. I know it's not your fault. I know you've given me thousands of dollars. You don't have to come out here. . . . Just love me, Daddy."

What Arnold apparently is hearing from Daddy is a lecture. "I know Daddy, I know. . . . You're right. . . . You're right. Daddy, that's not what I need to hear right now." He starts crying again.

All of a sudden, Arnold blurts out: "Daddy, can I be buried in the family plot at the cemetery? Next to Mom and

you? . . . Oh, thank you, Daddy. That sounds so good.
. . ."

The conversation goes on for longer than I expected.
When Arnold hangs up, I ask him how it went.

"Well, he lectured me on how I've lived my life. And I
agreed with him. Then he started crying, and I knew then
that he loved me. That's all I need to know."

If we know we are truly loved and not abandoned, we
can face the fear of death. The pastoral task as death draws
near to those we love is to represent Emmanuel—*God with
us.*

There is an eternal truth in the Christian doctrine of the
Incarnation: Jesus, though divine in nature, shared our human
nature "so that by his death he might destroy him who holds
the power of death . . . and free those who all their lives were
held in slavery by their fear of death" (Heb. 2:14-15).

Likewise, the doctrine of the Resurrection is more than a
metaphor of hope: Christ has indeed been raised from the
dead, and is alive today by God's Spirit! If Jesus Christ has
not been raised, our faith is futile. This truth is a sign to all
that the dead in Christ shall be raised to new life. We will
not remain asleep; we will be changed "in a flash, in the
twinkling of an eye, at the last trumpet" (I Cor. 15:52). The
Apostle Paul goes on to say that when death has been
swallowed up in victory, the hope of the prophet Hosea
will ring true:

I will ransom them from the power of the grave;
    I will redeem them from death.
Where, O death, are your plagues?
    Where, O grave, is your destruction? (Hos. 13:14)

Belief in a resurrection and overcoming the fear of death
are spiritual comforts that must be appropriated as matters

of personal faith. Truth cannot be imposed or transferred one to another. However, pastoral and professional care-givers aware of the *acceptance* stage of death and dying can encourage patients to face their own mortality. Once a person accepts the inevitability of death, a care-giver can be active in the final tasks of that person's life.

PREPARING TO DIE

As a terminally ill patient begins to accept the reality that death is coming, there will be things to do, places to visit, and people to see in order to get ready to die. This is called *taking care of business.* As discussed in chapter 7, the patient may want to be forgiven for failures in the past, reconcile with family and friends in the present, make peace with God, with the church, and with himself or herself for the future. The patient may have an unfinished project to complete or other internal or relational work to do. Encourage the patient to take care of any unfinished business.

Besides completing life tasks, there are practical arrangements that must be made. It may be helpful to discuss what desires your patient might have for his or her funeral and burial.

Philosophically and spiritually, patients during the final stage may continue asking themselves ultimate questions: "Have I made a contribution to life? Have I completed what I am here to do? Will I be remembered after I'm gone? What will happen after I die?" Pastors and care-givers cannot answer these questions concretely, but we can talk about them with our patients. People with terminal illnesses usually reach a point where they are no longer calling for healing power to recover; they are *answering the Light.* At this point, the appropriate task—for care-givers, family, friends, and all concerned—is to give permission to let go, to cross over, and to move toward the Light.

Giving permission is never easy, especially for family members. It means committing and releasing a person into the hands of God. It means losing control of the relationship and trusting in the possibilities of the great unknown. As difficult as it is, granting permission is important for both you and your patient. The value for you is that *you* need closure. Some kind of completion is necessary before *you* can move on. The value for your patient is that he or she needs permission to die. Patients may hold on and delay dying for the sake of a friend or family member they hate to leave behind. "There is a time for every purpose under heaven," and when the time comes for a person to die, we must detach ourselves. The one we love has suffered enough, is being called to the next life, and is trying to answer the Light.

Saying good-bye is a good way to grant permission to a patient who is ready to die. The process happens both verbally and non-verbally in the dynamic of the moment. To say good-bye requires preparing yourself outside the room for what you need to do and say inside the room during what may be your last visit. Look your patient directly in the eyes. Tell your patient how you feel: "I'm afraid that I won't see you again. . . . I've really valued our times together. I really appreciate you (or love you). I'm going to miss you. Good-bye, my friend."

The person to whom you are bidding farewell may or may not be able to respond. Nevertheless, the person will hear you, and the message will get through: "It's okay, I am free to go."

Once you say good-bye, you may or may not want to linger. Whether you personally remain for the duration, or someone else relieves you, the truth remains: *No one should have to die alone!*

Not everyone will die a calm and peaceful death. Some will quietly expire, often in the company of someone they love. Others will hang on seemingly forever and choose to die alone in the middle of the night. People usually die the way they live their lives. The quality of one's death often reflects the quality of one's life at the end stage. Unresolved, angry persons often die confused and enraged. Those who have made peace with the past, present, and future, who have resolved their issues, reconciled their relationships, and completed their work, often die in peace and dignity. There is some choice involved in how we die, and there is an ideal way to leave this life. As Mother Teresa says, "The greatest aim in human life is to die in peace with God."

Letting God Be God
by Barb Rost

I live in a suburb of Chicago, and I was afraid to travel to San Francisco to visit my brother, Ron, who was dying of AIDS. I feared both the city and what Ron would look like when I saw him.

My parents both are gone, and my brother is my only flesh and blood relative. I am married with four children, and belong to Chicago First Church of the Nazarene.

My brother became a Christian in 1982 and left the gay life-style. He showed definite and exciting evidence of spiritual life and growth in Christ for about two years. Besides being active in church, he underwent extensive counseling in an ex-gay ministry. However, this issue was a continual struggle for him, and he gradually went back into a gay life-style and moved to San Francisco.

I had just about given up on my brother, until he told me he had AIDS.

At first he said not to come out; he didn't want to see me. I called Michael Christensen in San Francisco and asked him to visit Ron in the hospital. Michael made two visits and encouraged me to come out and stay a while and seek reconciliation.

Ron was sleeping when I walked into his hospital room. I woke him, and the words came easily:

"I love you, Ron."

He told me he loved me, too.

"I want to ask you something, Ron. If ever in my life as a sister I have been insensitive to you and your needs; if ever I have not been the sister I should be, I want to ask you to forgive me."

Ron asked the same of me, and we had a marvelous reunion and reconciliation as family. I stayed for twelve days as his condition continued to deteriorate.

I had prayed for Christians to surround and uphold me in San Francisco during my visit. I stayed at the Care House—the Golden Gate Ministries hospitality house—and received tremendous support from Clark and Nancy, who manage it. But most of my time was spent with Ron and his friends, a very unexpected blessing.

Ron's friends were gay, and I had never been around gay people besides my brother. Before my trip to San Francisco, when I thought of homosexuals, I thought of militants who march, who are angry, who demand rights and laws passed. My attitudes changed when I got to know Ron's friends as individuals. They were very kind to me. They came to church with me, and I was able to share my faith in Jesus Christ with three of my brother's closest friends.

Ron remained hospitalized, and I returned home for two weeks. Leaving Ron was one of the most difficult things I have ever done! When I left Ron, I was crying and told him to hold on until I could get back to him. My four small children needed me. I would tend to them and then come back. I did everything but give him permission to die. Perhaps he was ready, but it was obvious that I was not.

179

I returned to San Francisco because I very much wanted to be with my brother when he died. Every night after visiting him, I prayed to the Lord: "Please let me be with Ron when he dies." I really agonized over this.

After the third day, God began speaking to me about this request. I felt him saying, "Let me decide what is best." Although there was nothing wrong with my desire to be with my brother until the end, I felt that the spiritual theme of my visit was "Let God be God."

I shared this new attitude, based on what God was showing me, with Ron's friends and his doctor. I can't tell you what peace came over me when I committed the *timing* of Ron's death to God.

I asked the Lord to show me if Ron had any spiritual life left in him. In the course of my visit, there were certain things he did and said to let me know he still had faith. I found Ron's Bible that Mom and Dad had given him when he became a Christian. I flipped through it and saw that he had underlined many passages. In the margin next to one verse about dying to sin, Ron wrote "Help me to understand this, Father." He called God *Father!* There's a lot that I don't understand about homosexuality and my brother's spirituality, but I was determined to "let God be God."

On the day I was scheduled to leave, the doctor told me Ron would probably die very soon, maybe that day. As much as I wanted it to happen during my visit, I needed to go home as planned. Actually, I felt in my heart that the Lord was lovingly saying no to my request to be present at Ron's death. Perhaps this dramatic change in me would be a positive witness to Ron's friends and the doctor.

Michael Christensen counseled me to say good-bye to Ron in such a way that let my brother know it was okay to die. I told him that I just couldn't tell my brother to let go; that sounds like I don't want him to live. Michael tried to explain the concept of granting permission, and I agreed to try it.

I stood over Ron in bed, looked him straight in the eyes, but there was no way I could tell him to let go. But I knew I was leaving, and I knew this was good-bye. The Lord helped me say it, and the words came easily.

Ron was unable to speak anymore, but I knew he could see me, and I knew he would understand. I got down close to Ron's face. Calmly, with love and compassion, but without any tears, I said: "Ron, I love you. I'm going to be leaving now. I'm going to the airport and probably won't see you again. I am so glad you are my brother. And I know you can't talk to me. I'm sure that must be frustrating, so I'll talk for you. I know you love me and are glad I'm your sister.

"You are going to be in heaven soon, and you'll be with the Lord. There will be no more pain or suffering or struggles. And you're going to see Mom and Dad again. I'm envious of that. When you see Mom and Dad, will you tell them I love them, too?"

I gave my brother a kiss, brushed his cheek with my hand, and went out the door. I turned around and gave Ron one last look and final good-bye: "I love you Ron, and I'll see you in heaven."

From behind the curtain, I watched Ron's eyes roll back in his head, until there was only white. He was unconscious. I wanted to stay for the duration; yet, I wanted to "let God be God."

I got back home to Chicago about six hours later. When I called the hospital, they told me Ron had just died. They said he never regained consciousness after I left. The Lord worked it out perfectly, for although I was not with him at the moment of death, I was with him for his last moment of consciousness. I was glad I allowed God to be God.

PASTORAL CARE AT THE TIME OF DEATH

"There is a time to be born and a time to die" the Scriptures affirm. As a minister or care-giver, you will be expected to know what to do at the time of death. Professional and pastoral care are especially needed by family and friends gathered at the deathbed and at the funeral or memorial service.

Ministry at the Deathbed

A person with AIDS whom you have been in contact with is dying or has just died, and you are summoned to the deathbed. What do you say and do when you can't resurrect the dead? As much as you would prefer to be spontaneous, it is better to think through in advance how best to respond. Having a definite plan or program in mind will enhance the quality of your spiritual help at the time of death.

The program I use and recommend consists of three parts: (1) recalling the facts, (2) offering a closure ritual (sometimes called Last Rites), and (3) reading prayers of farewell.

(1) *Recalling the facts* is simply compassionate conversation with family and friends about what is happening or has happened: How close is this person to death? How and when did this person die? Who was here when it happened? How are you doing at the moment? A profoundly painful and powerful event is occuring or has just occurred, and the people involved have a need to tell the story to a professional care-giver or clergy.

(2) *A closure ritual* is called for during the death process or soon after a person has died. The ritual acts as a catharsis experience to complete a life on earth. We symbolize our remembrance so that we ourselves may be healed. We enact a rite of passage to give family and friends an opportunity to relieve emotions. Through liturgy and involvement we have access to spiritual resources, which bring joy in the midst of sorrow. Closure rituals facilitate the transition from death to new life.

A simple ritual of closure is to touch and anoint the deceased with oil, ask the Spirit to accompany the departed on his or her journey home, and recite the ancient prayer of commendation:

Depart, O Christian soul, out of this world;
In the Name of God the Father Almighty who created you;
In the Name of Jesus Christ who redeemed you;
In the Name of the Holy Spirit who sanctifies you.
May your rest be this day in peace,
    and your dwelling place in the Paradise of God.[1]

This prayer can be prayed before or after a person has died. When family and friends are present, they should be invited to participate in the ritual. You might have them light candles or play meditative music. Invite them to gather around the body and read appropriate passages of Scripture.

(3) *Prayers of farewell* are the most important part of ministry at the time of death. People will look to you, as a minister or care-giver, to initiate a time of prayer. Start by offering thanks for this person who is dying or has died. Affirm the person's life and gifts and calling, yet speak the truth. Don't ignore the failure, pain, and loss. Say what is real and true without judgment.

Invite others to add their prayers and thoughts to what you have said. Ask family members, "Is there something you would like to say to God about this person?" Wait at least two minutes. People are often reluctant to pray, to surface their thoughts and intentions. People who are not accustomed to verbal prayer, if given permission, will verbalize their thoughts directly to the dying or deceased

---

[1] From the *Book of Common Prayer*. This may be adapted to more generic and inclusive forms, depending on the person's faith tradition or lack thereof. The *Book of Common Prayer* is a useful tool in ministry.

person as well as to God in prayer. Close by asking God to help and bless us all in the days of grief ahead, and invite everyone to join together in praying the Lord's Prayer. Almost everyone knows the Lord's Prayer and probably will feel good about praying it in this important, sacramental moment. Don't be afraid of being too religious in the aftermath of death. Death and dying is a sacred rite of passage.

"In My Father's House Are Many Rooms"

As a chaplain, I have had the privilege of being with several people with AIDS before and after their deaths. How vividly I remember the day my friend Daniel died.

It was Thursday afternoon, and I was making my rounds at General Hospital. My office had me paged on the AIDS ward. "Daniel died, and Martin is trying to reach you." Quickly, I called Martin. He was in a panic: "Well, it happened; the body is still here; can you come?" I said I would be right there.

En route to the home of Martin and Daniel, I reflect on the year and a half I have known these two gay men and been involved in their lives. I remember the shock I felt when Daniel, at thirty-five years of age, was diagnosed with AIDS. He and I were the same age—too young to die! I remember the courage and dignity with which Daniel dealt with his diagnosis, how inspired I was by his desire to live every day to its fullest.

I recall the joy of sitting in a coffee house with his partner, Martin, as he prayed the prayer I taught him—"Lord Jesus Christ, have mercy on me a sinner." On the day that Martin took his own HIV blood test, before knowing the outcome of the test, he had a spiritual breakthrough.

I remember the many conversations I had with Daniel, both at his home and at the outpatient clinic at General. I especially remember the last conversation I had with him just a few days prior to his death. He had shared with me the joy of letting go and preparing to die. He told me all his tasks were completed, his bags were packed, and he was ready to go home. He rejoiced that he had spent time with his family and made peace with his father. He said he had seen glimpses of the other side where God was waiting for him. "I'm going to miss you, Daniel!" I said as I embraced him. He thanked me for being his pastor. I thanked him for being my teacher in the school of death and dying. And then we said good-bye.

Daniel stayed alive for another week. When I arrived at his home on the day he died, three friends surrounded his bed, waiting for something to happen that would signal release. I asked them to tell me how he died.

Martin told me about Daniel's remark the other night that seemed incoherent: "I don't know about this room they keep talking about. It's green, not red." I reminded him of Jesus' statement about heaven: "In my Father's house are many rooms" (John 14:2).

Martin and his friend Amy told me about how Daniel summoned them that morning, saying: "I'm going to die today. I love you; I love you all." As Martin described it, "Daniel's eyes rolled inward, he looked the other way, his gaze shifted to what was waiting for him on the other shore."

Daniel Brewer, who would have turned thirty-six later in the month, died quietly and peacefully at home, surrounded by those he loved.

I suggested we anoint Daniel's body with oil and commend him to God. The lights were dimmed. A candle was lit, I read some scriptures and asked everyone to pray a simple, heartfelt prayer. Using oil, I made the sign of the cross on Daniel's cold brow and recited the ancient words of commendation: "Depart O Christian Soul. . . . "

When all was said and done, the candle was extinguished, we hugged one another and left the room. The mortician was waiting patiently outside. I helped him lift the six-foot-four-inch, rigid body onto the gurney and carry it down the stairs and into the van. Martin could not bear to look at his partner wrapped in a plastic bag.

Courageously, Martin made arrangements for cremation and the funeral. The Requiem Mass at Grace Cathedral was as eclectic as Daniel's faith and spirituality. There were scriptures read, poems recited, and eulogies delivered. A black gospel choir sang "I Surrender All"—echoing the process Daniel had gone through in letting go and preparing to die. The Eucharist was offered in high Anglican style by the Dean of the Cathedral and me. The service ended with the congregation singing the stately hymn "O Jerusalem":

Bring me my coat of finest gold
Bring me mine arrows of desire
Bring me my shield of power and might
Bring me my chariots of fire
I shall not cease the blessed fight
Nor shall my sword sleep in mine hand
'till thee I see Jerusalem
'neath England's sweet and precious light.

I mourn the loss of my friend Daniel, for I had grown to love him and respect his faith. I thank God he did not have to die alone, but at home, surrounded by those he loved. The pain was minimal. He did not gasp for breath, resist the process, or "rage against the dying of the light." Instead, he expired gracefully, dignified to the very end. And God *was* waiting for him on the other shore.

Participating in a Funeral Service

Sometimes AIDS care-givers are called upon to conduct or participate in a funeral or memorial service. The same three-part program previously discussed—*recalling the*

186

facts, offering a closure ritual, and *leading prayers of farewell*—can be adapted for such a purpose.

At a funeral or memorial service, *recalling the facts* would take the form of a eulogy celebrating a person's life and acknowledging his or her death. The occasion calls for both seriousness and humor. People need permission to laugh and cry.

The *closure ritual* is the heart of the funeral ceremony and should have both formal and informal elements. The same needs for closure that are present at the deathbed resurface at the funeral: emotional catharsis, completion of a life on earth, remembrance that allows healing, an opportunity for family and friends to express themselves, and an occasion to access spiritual resources and facilitate the transition.

Prayers of farewell may be offered by clergy, family members, and friends. It is good to invite those present to share a remembrance of the departed in the atmosphere of prayer. Remembering the departed and the needs of those left behind is a fitting form of prayer. Offering our thoughts and prayers in silence is also a meaningful way to complete a life at a funeral service.

When a person dies, there are many edifying and truthful things that can be said, and there is at least one thing that should never be said. *Never* say or imply to family and friends gathered to mourn the loss of someone who has died of AIDS—"It must have been God's will." It is not in the compassionate nature of God to will the tragic or premature death of anyone. As William Sloane Coffin, renowned former minister of Riverside Church in New York City, preached at his own son's death:

> God doesn't go around this world with his finger on triggers, his fist around knives, his hands on steering wheels. . . . My own consolation lies in knowing that it

was not the will of God that Alex die; that when the waves closed over the sinking car, God's heart was the first to break.

It is important to help family and friends understand at the funeral that God deplores disease and unnatural death. It is *not* God's will for people to die of AIDS. Yes, actions have consequences; sexual carelessness and drug abuse increase one's risk of AIDS, and "the wages of sin is death." These things are true. But in theology and pastoral care, we must not attribute tragedy and disease to the direct will and intention of God. While natural death at a ripe old age is a part of life, dying in pain and agony in the prime of one's life is always horrific. In this era of AIDS, tragedies will continue to occur and Jesus' tears are the first to be shed.

FACING YOUR OWN MORTALITY

The surest way to become a compassionate and effective care-giver when death draws near is to *face your own mortality*. Those who have faced their own death can teach others about the Light at the end of the tunnel. Those who have not dealt with their own death will perpetuate society's avoidance of this dark and awkward subject.

The first step in looking at death is to realize that *the worse could happen to me!*

The Worse Can Happen to Me

From the time of our youth we delude ourselves into thinking that we are invincible: Others get sick, but I probably will not. Others have accidents, but not me. Others lose their money and source of livelihood, but nothing like that could ever happen to me. Members of other's families get into trouble, are caught breaking the law, are sentenced to prison, suffer divorce, but I will experience no such misfortune. Others may be forced to stand by and watch their loved ones get cancer or AIDS, suffer and die, but God will protect me and my family from such calamity.

In times of health and happiness we must remember that God has promised us no physical or temporal immunities, and that the worse may happen to any of us.

I read a powerful devotional reflection on this subject by James B. Chapman, an early formative influence on the Church of the Nazarene. He cautions Christians, especially those who claim a special relationship with God, not to presume that the worst-case scenario will not occur:

Today my car may be wrecked, my fortune may fly away, my position may fold up, my child may sicken, my health may permanently fail, my dearest friend may die—I may die myself. . . .

And if no calamity comes, even then I must not take this good fortune to mean that God is smiling on me. God sends His sun to shine on the righteous as well as the unrighteous, and causes rain to fall on good and bad alike. . . .

Exterior circumstances—either poverty or prosperity— are not sufficient evidence of God's favor or judgment. . . .

He has not promised immunity to passing sorrow, but has promised that joy shall follow sorrow. . . . He has not promised that our mines shall yield nothing but gold; but He has promised that we ourselves shall come out of the furnace as refined as gold. He has not promised that we shall not be separated from our loved ones; but He has promised that we shall be united with our loved ones after the separation. . . . He has not promised that we ourselves shall not grow old, sicken and die; but He has promised that we shall arise in eternal and painless youth. . . .

Therefore, even though the worst that can come to

mortals may come to me, I shall yet have the best that comes to immortals in full compensation, and I shall be glad forever.[2]

Visualizing Your Own Death

A second step in facing personal mortality is to envision your own death. Take an imaginative journey through an AIDS diagnosis, through the onset of symptoms, to the actual death experience, and beyond. Try to picture your own funeral and burial. Reflect on who is there and what they are saying about you. Read the epitaph on your tombstone. What is the one line that summarizes your life?

This is not intended to be a morbid exercise, but a creative way of dealing with one's own mortality. For those of us who have never had a near-death experience, visualizing one's death is a method to stimulate terminal illness might involve.

The following "Death Personalization Exercise" is conducted by Shanti Project, a leading AIDS services provider in San Francisco. It is offered to chaplains and care-givers at General Hospital as part of their basic training. It is most deeply experienced when you are relaxed and reflective, and when someone else slowly reads you the following suggestions:

Several weeks ago, you noticed a small purplish spot on your right leg. At first, you thought it looked like a bruise. It didn't itch like an insect bite. It reminded you of pictures you had seen of KS lesions. You remembered receiving blood several years ago and begin to worry it may have brought you AIDS. A growing sense of concern and worry come over you. You decide to make an appointment with your doctor to settle the question.

---

[2] J. B. Chapman, "The Worse Can Happen to Me," *Religion and Everyday Life*, (Kansas City: Beacon Hill Press, 1945), pp. 19-21. Used by permission.

(Pause)

During your examination, your doctor finds several swollen lymph glands. Tissue samples from the glands are taken, and a series of tests are done. Imagine what it is like waiting in the doctor's office and examination rooms.

(Pause 30 seconds)

Four days later, the doctor's nurse calls and says, "We have the results of the test, and the doctor would like to see you as soon as possible about them." What feelings do you experience as you hang up the phone and get ready to go to your doctor's office?

(Pause 30 seconds)

Now you're sitting in the doctor's office, and wondering what the test results will be. You sense that the usually friendly receptionist is avoiding looking at you.

(Pause)

What do you feel as the doctor enters, says hello, and proceeds to inform you that you have a severe case of Kaposi's Sarcoma? You have AIDS. Your doctor says you have many lesions inside your body and tells you of your treatment options. Your doctor tells you your life expectancy is less than a year, speaking with the overtone of anxious despair. Do you say anything to your doctor before leaving his office?

(Pause 30 seconds)

You leave the office and return home. You feel a strange numbness in your body, and your mind is trying to make sense of what's happening.

Allow yourself to notice the thoughts and experience the feelings and sensations that arise in your body, as you wonder what to do now. Where do you go? To whom do you turn?

(Pause 1 minute)

Time passes.

(Pause)

As you recover from the initial shock, you begin the painful process of telling the significant people in your life. How do people respond to your illness: your family, your children, your friends, your roommates, your co-workers? One-by-one, picture each significant person in your life and imagine *their* response to learning you have AIDS.

(Pause 2 minutes)

Are there any persons you decide not to tell? If so, why?

(Pause 1 minute)

Who will most likely be close to you at this time, and who will be most afraid and withdraw? Who will be most open to you and your needs? Picture your parents, children, brothers and sisters, lover, and friends. What feelings do *you* have about each person as you imagine them drawing closer or pulling away?

(Pause 1 minute)

Time passes.

(Pause)

Four months have passed. You have responded well to treatment and consider yourself to be in fairly good health. One day you begin to notice a shortness of breath. You develop a dry cough and high fever. Almost overnight you find yourself in the hospital being treated for pneumocystis pneumonia, an infection of the lungs. Imagine how you feel about this sudden change in your situation.

(Pause 1 minute)

While in the hospital, you wake up one morning feeling confused and disoriented. The last few days are full of vague recollections of painful procedures. You wonder what's been happening to you. What do you feel as you ponder this question: "What's going to happen next?"

(Pause 30 seconds)

By the time the pneumocystis pneumonia is effectively treated, you have eighty lesions on the surface of your body. Many are on your face. You sometimes feel that people look more at your lesions than at you. Despite your ongoing attempts to stay positive, at times you feel it's too much to bear. How do you handle feeling so helpless and vulnerable?

(Pause 1 minute)

How has AIDS affected the amount of affection you give and receive?

(Pause)

What effect has it had on your sensuality and expression?

(Pause 1 minute)

You now more frequently feel that you are dying. How has AIDS altered your life's goals and dreams? What emotions arise in trying to live your remaining life?

(Pause 1 minute)

As you lie awake at night, unable to sleep, imagine yourself thinking about these questions:

"What has been the purpose of my life?"

"What is the meaning of it now?"

"Am I satisfied with this meaning?"

(Pause 1 minute)

Over a year has passed since you heard the diagnosis in your doctor's office. You have become progressively weaker and are feeling very sick now. You have become so sick that you need to be admitted to a hospital. You know that there is limited time remaining. Call each significant person in your life, one-by-one, into your room. Say anything you'd like to each one, anything you may have left unsaid, anything you want to repeat. Imagine each person's words to you. Then, one-by-one, say good-bye to all the people you love and who love you.

(Pause 2 minutes)

You are feeling very tired now. Just moving seems to take monumental effort, and suddenly you begin to feel that it is time to die.

Behind you there is a light through which is visible a familiar scene. Doctors and nurses are working over a body trying to bring it back to life. You see that the body was once yours. What do you feel as you observe their efforts? Do you want them to succeed?

(Pause 30 seconds)

As you realize that they have not been able to revive you, what do

193

you observe being done to, and with, your body? Is this what you would want done?

(Pause 30 seconds)

Imagine yourself standing at the opening of a lighted tunnel. Enter the tunnel and proceed at your own pace, as quickly or as slowly as you like. As you go through the tunnel try to observe what it is like and what emotions you are feeling as you go on your journey.

(Pause 1 minute)

What are the next events to take place? Is there a memorial service, a cremation, a burial?

(Pause 30 seconds)

If there is a service, what are your feelings as you listen to the words chosen to describe your life? Do you feel that they truly represent you?

(Pause 45 seconds)

What do you experience as you observe the faces of the mourners present? Is there anybody who isn't there whom you expected to attend?

(Pause 1 minute)

Now that the memorial service is at an end, what awaits you on your journey through the tunnel?

(Pause 1 minute)

This exercise is now at an end, and the picture before you is fading. As the light dims, realize that this has been an exercise. Take as much time as you need to return to your body, to this room, to the present and, when you are ready, open your eyes.

When all your group is ready, share within your group what this experience has been like for you.[3]

---

[3]*Shanti Project* is a non-profit organization currently providing free volunteer-based support services to people with AIDS/disabling HIV disease and their families, friends, and loved ones in San Francisco. Services include practical and emotional support, staff counseling at SF General Hospital, a residence program, and an activities program for people with AIDS and disabling HIV.

In experiencing this vivid exercise, we realize our mortality and face our fear of death. By visualizing our own death, we prepare ourselves and are prepared for others to cross over. The quality of pastoral care at the time of death is enhanced by remembering how mortal we are and finding our hope in God.

For all who believe and hope in God, there is Light at the end of the tunnel. As we walk through the valley of the shadow of death with people with AIDS, we do not have to be afraid,

for Thou art with me. Thy rod and thy staff, they comfort me. Thou preparest a table before me in the presence of my enemies: thou anointest my head with oil; my cup runneth over. Surely goodness and mercy shall follow me all the days of my life: and I will dwell in the house of the Lord forever. (Ps. 23:4-6 KJV)

195

CHAPTER TEN

AIDS Is a Word from God—
Are We Listening?

"God is speaking to us through this disease."

A few weeks before Easter I was visiting Ray, a patient at Mother Teresa's AIDS home in San Francisco. Ray was raised in the Russian Orthodox church and had a beautiful shrine next to his bed complete with candles, icons, incense, and an open Bible. His faith was evident in his eyes. Though his body was weak, Ray had grown strong in spirit. For him, AIDS had been a healing agent of God, calling him to take stock of his life, receive forgiveness and strength, and be renewed in the faith of his childhood. The result of the AIDS crisis for him was spiritual restoration and peace with his Creator. All things were made new.

On the morning that I was visiting Ray, Mother Teresa was also visiting the house, and Ray had the chance to meet her. Although I could not hear their conversation, I knew her way of pastoral care and her view of AIDS.

Mother Teresa's spirit is not judgmental but rather unconditionally loving and fully present. She sees the whole person as a child of God and does not focus on a person's sins or how a disease is contracted. She also sees within a suffering person the suffering presence of Christ and is grateful for the opportunity to serve Jesus by serving someone with AIDS.

Mother Teresa's view of AIDS is based on a spiritual

understanding that *AIDS is a word from God*. "God is speaking to us through this disease," she told a group of volunteers who visited her in Calcutta. If Mother Teresa is right about AIDS being a word *from* God, rather than a judgment *of* God, then what is God saying? Reflecting on this insight, I hear at least three words.

THE FIRST WORD—TO THE PERSON WITH AIDS

The first word is heard by the person with a terminal disease: get ready for a crisis! The Chinese written character for *crisis* means *opportunity* for good or evil.

AIDS is a tragedy; yet, there is within the crisis the inherent opportunity for AIDS to be the agent of healing and bridge of hope to the God of all comfort and light. Chronic illness can lead to redemption. Suffering can force us to search the depths of our soul where we find strength, hope, and God's healing presence. Terminal illness can be the agent that connects us to our compassionate Creator. How a person is able to process the disease and draw on the spiritual resources within or from the ministry of others will determine the outcome of the crisis.

We may find God in AIDS, but we may also be defeated by suffering, become embittered toward life, and shut out the healing presence of God. AIDS is sometimes interpreted as a harsh word of wrath. How often I hear people say: "God is punishing me" or "I guess I'm getting what I deserve." Persons with AIDS are usually very hard on themselves, and they don't need others to confirm their guilt or the anger they feel from God. What they need to hear is that the "Lord is compassionate and gracious, slow to anger and abounding in love" (Ps. 103:8). They need to know that God is the One "who forgives all your sins and heals all your diseases, who redeems your life from the pit and crowns you with love and compassion" (Ps. 103:4).

They need to be surrounded by those who love and support them as they complete unfinished business in their lives and receive God's provisions.

For the person with AIDS who is able to see the brighter hope of ultimate good behind the cloud of suffering, AIDS presents an opportunity to look within oneself and to draw nearer to God. In the light of love and forgiveness, one can take stock of life—one's failures and successes, transitions and triumphs, paths and destinations.

If you are a person with AIDS, consider it a part of your personal pilgrimage. Ask yourself, what do I need to complete before I die? What unfinished business do I have? Who do I need to see, talk to, or be reconciled with? Begin setting your affairs in order by reconciling your relationships and completing any unfinished tasks. As life and breath are given, enjoy every moment. Live deeply, intentionally, and fully. As death approaches, prepare to leave everything behind. Make peace with God and with yourself.

Hearing God's word of grace involves deep repentance, transformation, and spiritual renewal. It sometimes involves the need for repentance. It sometimes involves changing one's ways, giving up control, and surrendering to "the God of all comfort" (II Cor. 1:3). Though it may involve sacrifice and sorrow, the terrible news of AIDS can bring a life-giving word from God.

THE SECOND WORD—TO THE CHURCH

The second word I hear in the AIDS crisis is a challenge for the Church to be the Church and respond with compassion. Compassion withholds judgment and opens its heart. Compassion allows your heart to be broken by that which breaks the heart of God. Compassion is basic in a ministry of presence, embracing the pain of another and mediating Christ's power to comfort and heal.

A compassionate response to people with AIDS is more concerned with the ministry of healing than in preserving moral doctrine. Whenever there is a choice between pastoral care and canon law (protecting church standards), always opt for pastoral care. People matter more than doctrines! This is especially true with the controversial issues related to AIDS ministry.

The internationally known and respected Roman Catholic priest and scholar Henri Nouwen writes in *The Road to Daybreak* about his impressions of the gay district of San Francisco and the real issues in pastoral care:

> As I walked with my friend on the streets of the Castro district, we saw countless men walking up and down the sidewalks just looking at each other, gazing into store windows, standing on corners in small groups, and going in and out of bars, theaters, video shops, drugstores, and restaurants. It seemed as if everyone was waiting for something that would bring them a sense of being deeply loved, fully accepted, and truly at home. But evident in the eyes of the many was deep suffering, anguish, and loneliness, because what they most seek and most desire seems most elusive. Many have not been able to find a lasting home or a safe relationship, and now, with the AIDS threat, fear has become all-pervasive. . . .
>
> More than ever the Church has to live out Christ's love for the poor, the sinners, the publicans, the rejected, the possessed, and all who desperately need to be loved. As I saw countless gay men on the streets, I kept thinking about the great consolation that Jesus came to offer. He revealed the total and unlimited love of God for humanity. This is the love that the Church is called to make visible, not by judging, condemning, or segregating, but by serving everyone in need. I often wonder if the many heated debates about the morality of homosexuality do not prevent the Christian community from reaching out fearlessly to its suffering fellow humans (p. 200).

It is safer to *condemn* behavior and say, "People with AIDS get what they deserve!" It is more difficult to withhold our opinions and represent a God of comfort and tender mercies.

It took a little child living with AIDS and coming to church to convince me that AIDS is not a plague representing God's judgment. AIDS, I learned, is a disease that potentially could infect anyone.

It took heterosexuals living with AIDS and coming to church to convince me that AIDS is not a gay problem but a human challenge.

It took gay persons living with AIDS and coming to church to help me understand the meaning of God's unconditional love and acceptance of all whose hearts are open. They have taught me how to love and accept diversity in the Body of Christ, and not to put restrictions on God's grace.

It took recovering drug addicts and alcoholics living with AIDS and coming to church to show me that although actions have consequences, inner healing is possible. There is deliverance from compulsion and restoration from damaged emotions. There is forgiveness for the sin of injuring yourself or others.

A dramatic change in attitude takes place deep within our spirit when we get to know someone with AIDS. A miracle of transformation occurs when we hear and respond to the word from God challenging us to overcome our prejudice in brokenness and compassion.

THE THIRD WORD—TO THE DIVIDED HUMAN FAMILY

The third word I hear in AIDS is reconciliation. It is a word of hope for the outcast homosexual community and a word of challenge to the dominant heterosexual society. It is a word of peace and justice, an invitation to be forgiven of hatred, bigotry, separation from God, or self-righteousness, and together to be healed.

Jesus told a parable of a loving father and two sons. Either one could have been gay or have had AIDS. The one who squandered his money in the fast lane came to his senses and came home. The son who never left home was indignant and self-righteous. But the father rejoiced that his son "was dead and is now alive again; he was lost and now is found!" (Luke 16:24).

The attitude of the father is revealed in his outstretched hands and a heart of compassion that did not probe into the details of his son's life but simply forgave and celebrated the return home. As Henri Nouwen writes:

> God does not require a pure heart before embracing us. Even if we return only because following our desires has failed to bring happiness, God will take us back. Even if we return because being a Christian brings more peace than being a pagan, God will receive us. Even if we return because our sins did not offer as much satisfaction as we had hoped, God will take us back. Even if we return because we could not make it on our own, God will receive us. God's love does not require any explanations about why we are returning. God is glad to see us home and wants to give us all we desire, just for being home.[1]

God's word of reconciliation addressed to both gay and straight people in the broken and divided human family is simply "come home." Whether you remained within the boundaries of the church or not, "It's time to come home." No matter what the sin or separation, there is forgiveness at home. Gay or straight, saint or sinner, rebellious or obedient, infected or not infected, there is only one place of healing and love—*home* with God. Reconciliation is the

---

[1]*The Road to Daybreak* (New York: Doubleday, 1988), pp. 72-73.

road that leads to home. "Softly and tenderly," the word of God is being spoken. "Come home, come home, you who are weary, come home!"

There is a place in the kingdom of God for the outcasts and the diseased, including homosexuals and persons with AIDS. "In my father's house are many mansions," Jesus told us, and there's room enough for us all!

A PERSONAL WORD

"Why are you involved in AIDS ministry?" I am often asked. "Are you gay? Do *you* have AIDS? What attracts you to AIDS ministry more than homeless ministry or youth ministry? What do *you* get out of being an AIDS chaplain?"

To answer these questions requires some soul-searching. I believe that AIDS has a personal word from God for me. Upon reflection, I can identify six reasons I choose to minister as an AIDS chaplain.

1. *Personally*, AIDS has hit close to home. I have a gay cousin whose partner died with AIDS. Being with my cousin during his grief has challenged me to treat others as I would my own family.

2. *Spiritually*, I am attracted to AIDS ministry because I am called to follow a different path, to take the road less traveled and risk rejection. Perhaps I identify with outcast groups, like homeless persons and people with AIDS, in a way that I do not identify with those who are socially accepted and who fit the norm. I doubt that I have the gifts and aptitude for mainstream ministry.

3. *Psychologically*, AIDS ministry challenges my desire to be in control and provides opportunities for me to be vulnerable and depend totally on God. Visiting and supporting people with AIDS is an unpredictable experience during which there are no pat answers and almost

202

anything can happen. For ministers with control issues and difficulty admitting weakness, AIDS ministry reminds us that we are helpless in the face of this disease. Our only hope is in God and the healing that God brings.

As in all authentic ministry, when I let go of the need to control the outcome, I find that I receive greater gifts and blessings. I may offer comfort to someone in need, but what I gain in return is spiritual assurance that God is waiting for me when my time has come.

4. *Emotionally*, AIDS ministry engages my heart as no other ministry does. Expressing emotions does not come easily to me. I am attracted to the depth of emotions and breadth of feelings that are expressed around the issues of death and dying, pain and suffering, healing and transformation. To look into a person's eyes and see the spirit of Jesus, to receive the gifts that person has to offer, to reach out and hold the hand of someone ready to die, to be affirmed by people who are grateful for a care-giver, and to pray with someone who needs the touch of God are pastoral experiences that touch my own needs and feed my soul.

5. *Motivationally*, the "wounded healer" insight reveals why I minister. The story is told of twelve ministers and theologians of all faiths and twelve psychiatrists of all faiths convening for a two-day, off-the-record conference. "The chairman, a psychiatrist, opened the seminar with this question: 'We are all healers, whether we are ministers or doctors. Why are we in this business? What is our motivation?' There followed only ten minutes of intense discussion and they all agreed, doctors and ministers, Catholics, Jews, and Protestants. 'For our own healing,' they said" (from *Servant Leadership* by Robert Greenleaf).

I am not alone in finding healing for my own wounds and resolution of my own issues through the avenue of service to others. Christians are attracted to ministry—*for their own healing* as well as to help others. The primary reason God calls us into ministry is so that God can heal us. And in the process of our own healing, others are helped and healed.

6. *Finally*, I am attracted to AIDS ministry because of the joy and fulfillment it brings to me. As one who is interested in the mysteries of this life as well as the life hereafter, there is much I learn from those facing death. And there is deep joy caring for those so often neglected.

Important, life-changing things happen when I visit someone with AIDS. The moment I walk into a room wearing a clerical collar or a badge that says "chaplain" I can count on getting a reaction. I represent not only God but also the church, and all the positive or negative experiences a person in the hospital bed has accumulated over the years. It will all surface if I will but sit and listen. In being present to the depth of feeling and experience, without judging and without preaching, a spiritual connection is made that may last a lifetime. And in that very human connection and interaction, the suffering love and joyful presence of Christ is found.

To sense the spirit of Christ in human suffering, as well as the joy of his redeeming love, is one of the greatest gifts of compassionate ministry. Nothing in this world can compare with the challenging, captivating, cleansing experience of a heart warmed by divine presence. In the light of the holy, one can only feebly echo the mortal words of Isaiah: "I saw the Lord on a throne, high and exalted, and the train of his robe filled the temple. . . . Holy, holy, holy is the Lord Almighty, the whole earth is full of his glory" (Isa. 6:1, 3).

In the final years of this century, as the AIDS epidemic accelerates to its peak, I believe God is speaking to us all through this disease. God is speaking to the person with

AIDS, as well as to the church. God is speaking to the gay community as well as to mainstream society. And God is speaking to me personally.

Is God speaking to you, the reader of this book? I challenge you to look into your heart and offer what you find there. Buried beneath the surface of our lives there is a truth and calling awaiting its time of fulfillment. When you discern that personal message and calling, you must trust and obey at all costs. You may be rejected, and certainly misunderstood by those who do not share your truth and calling, but God's affirmation is what matters most.